Obstetric and Gynaecological Ultrasound Made Easy

Commissioning Editor: Ellen Green
Development Editor: Barbara Simmons
Project Manager: Emma Riley
Designer: Erik Bigland

Obstetric and Gynaecological Ultrasound Made Easy

Norman C. Smith MD FRCOG
Consultant Obstetrician and Honorary Senior Lecturer
Obstetric Ultrasound and Fetal Assessment Unit
Aberdeen Maternity Hospital
Aberdeen, UK

A. Pat M. Smith MD DRCOG PGCert Med Ed
Associate Specialist and Honorary Lecturer
Obstetric Ultrasound and Fetal Assessment Unit
Aberdeen Maternity Hospital
Aberdeen, UK

Second Edition

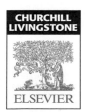

Edinburgh London New York Oxford Philadelphia St Louis Sydney Toronto 2006

Preface

There are many comprehensive texts on advanced obstetric and gynaecological ultrasound but very few simple, concise ones for those beginning their training. *Obstetric and Gynaecological Ultrasound Made Easy* will be useful to medical students, radiographers, midwives and doctors. It will serve as a practical pocket guide and quick reference text for core knowledge. However, the skill in the acquisition of good images only develops with hands-on experience for which there is no substitute. Prints of normality and abnormality are given which will help the interpretation of what is seen in real time. The correct interpretation of ultrasound imaging for the beginner requires supervision by an experienced trainer. The text has been written from our experience as trainers and the facts gleaned from recent textbooks which are recommended for reference and further reading. Points to remember conclude each section to act as an aide-mémoire and to read the day before that final exam.

N C Smith
A P M Smith

Acknowledgements

We wish to thank all the staff in our department who have provided the inspiration to write this book. Every second opinion they have sought from us has helped to formulate the concepts presented.

Contents

SECTION 1

Obstetrics

How to learn obstetric scanning

The machine and its controls

When you first set eyes on a scan machine, you will see that there is a screen, a transducer and a panel with weird and wonderful controls (Fig. 1.1). You will soon be ready for take-off, much sooner than you think because the manufacturers have progressively developed more user-friendly equipment. You no longer require to have a deep understanding of the principles of the physics of ultrasound but more a working knowledge of how the machine acquires an image

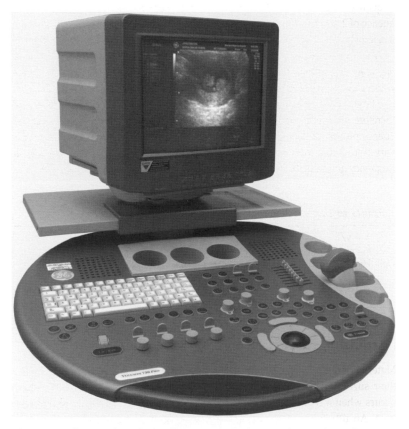

Fig. 1.1 *Ultrasound machine with screen, transducer and control panel.*

and how the controls can improve that image for you. A basic understanding of the different probes and how they transmit the ultrasound is also necessary.

Frequency and probes

Sound is a mechanical vibration distinguished by pitch (or frequency) and loudness. The velocity (v) of sound waves is constant (at 1540 m/s) and is determined by the wavelength (λ) multiplied by the frequency (f). Higher frequencies therefore mean that the wavelengths are shorter because the velocity is constant. The frequency is defined as the number of vibrations (or cycles) per second and the unit of frequency is termed Hertz (Hz) (cycles per second). Middle C on the piano has a frequency of 256 Hz and the octave above 512 Hz. Ultrasound is termed such because it cannot be heard by the human ear and has a frequency above 20 000 Hz (20 kHz).

The transducers on ultrasound machines have different frequencies and are in the range of 2–10 megahertz (MHz). Higher frequency probes have narrower beam widths and give better resolution which means they are more able to distinguish two targets close together. However, they have decreased penetration. You should therefore use higher frequency probes to visualise near structures and lower frequency probes for deeper structures. For obstetric scanning, the abdominal probes vary from 3 to 5 MHz and the transvaginal probes from 5 to 7.5 Hz, the higher frequency giving better resolution for structures close to the probe (Fig. 1.2).

Points to remember

1. $\lambda = v/f$.
2. f = cycles per second (Hz).
3. Higher frequency means narrower beam width, better resolution and poorer penetration.
4. Use higher frequency probes for near structures.

Acquisition of the image

Materials exist which produce an electric current when pressure is applied to their surface. This is known as the *piezoelectric effect* and the inverse effect occurs when a current is applied to the material causing it to expand and contract. An ultrasound transducer for pulse-echo imaging houses one or more slabs of piezoelectric material. An ultrasound pulse is generated and reflected from the target structures. The reflected echoes are then detected. This process is repeated in many directions to allow the target structures to be displayed on the screen. Present-day equipment employs *real-time imaging*, as opposed to static, and this provides an immediate image and reveals movement of the structures being examined. Most of the probes are now electronically rather than mechanically driven and utilise an *array system* which comprises scanned transducer elements mounted in line. Sets of elements are pulsed in sequence to produce a rectangular field of view. For obstetric use, curved array transducers are utilised (Fig. 1.2) which give a slightly wider field of view and are easier to manipulate on the lower abdomen in early pregnancy. Transvaginal probes work on the same principle.

The controls (Fig. 1.3)

You need to have a structured approach to obtain your best image on screen. You should be guided through the setting up of the machine by one of your friendly sonographers or, better still, a medical physicist who can also teach you a little science. Do not randomly twirl any knobs or press any keys to see if anything happens.

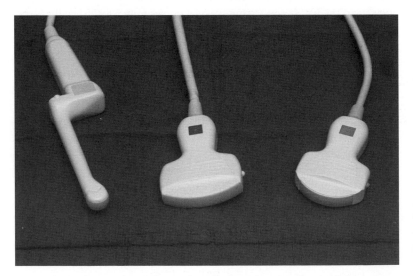

Fig. 1.2 *Various probes (left to right: transvaginal probe of variable frequency from 5 to 7.5 MHz, curvilinear probes 3.75 MHz and 5 MHz).*

1. **Where is the on–off switch?**

This is often hidden out of view of the control panel, sometimes at the side or back of the machine. Press the switch and the machine begins to hum and, in a few seconds, an outline of the image field appears on the screen.

2. **What probe do I use?**

It is likely that your medical physics department in liaison with the manufacturers have preset the machine for your convenience, utilising a probe preset key. Find it. Alternatively, there is likely to be a 'New Patient' key and when this is selected, the preset image will appear. You may have to make no further adjustments. In the first half of pregnancy, you will achieve good resolution and usually not require such deep penetration so a 5 MHz probe is satisfactory. Later in pregnancy, when a larger field is required with more penetration, a 3.5 MHz probe is better. For early pregnancy scanning, you must know the key to change to the transvaginal probe.

3. **Shall I adjust the brightness and contrast controls on the screen?**

You should not have to change these unless the previous user has been playing with them. These controls do not improve your scan and should not be changed

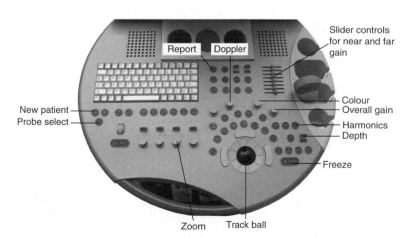

Fig. 1.3 Control panel.

during scanning. The brightness adjusts the screen background and the contrast alters the whiteness.

4. The field is not deep enough to view what I want.

You need to alter the *depth* control. You need to know this one because it requires frequent adjustment depending on the gestation and consequent fetal size. It is best to reduce depth as much as possible because this leads to a faster frame rate and better imaging. You can use the *zoom* control to expand an area of interest to fill the whole screen and modern machines do improve the quality of zoom. This is equivalent to using a zoom lens on your camera (Fig. 1.4).

5. The image is not all that good. Is there anything else I can do to improve it?

You may wish to adjust the *gain*. This changes the sensitivity to received echoes. Increasing the gain increases the echoes throughout the field and thus may improve the image where obesity is causing attenuation.

It may be that the images deep in the field are poor but the structures near the surface are clearer to see. You can alter small segments of the image to adjust for acoustic loss deeper in the field (*time gain compensation*). There are usually slider controls or individual knobs for such near or far gain control.

You may wish to adjust the *focal zone* to incorporate your area of interest. The beam is adjusted for optimum resolution at a particular distance from the probe and this occurs automatically with the probe selected. The focal zone is marked at the side of the screen (Fig. 1.4) and you can therefore see where it is in relation to your area of interest and focus accordingly.

If you are scanning an obese patient you may wish to adjust the tissue *harmonics*. This option has become available in recent equipment. The receiver amplifier is tuned to a centre frequency which is twice that of the transmission pulse. By doing this, weak transmission pulses such as those in the beam's side lobes, and those due to reverberation and multiple scattering are eliminated. This results in a reduction in sensitivity and axial resolution and so is not useful in thin patients.

There is still more (if you are a controls freak) but further refinement of your image for basic obstetric ultrasound scanning will not be required. On a note of caution, avoid increasing acoustic power because this exposes the fetus to more ultrasound and will have been set already by the manufacturer or your medical physics department.

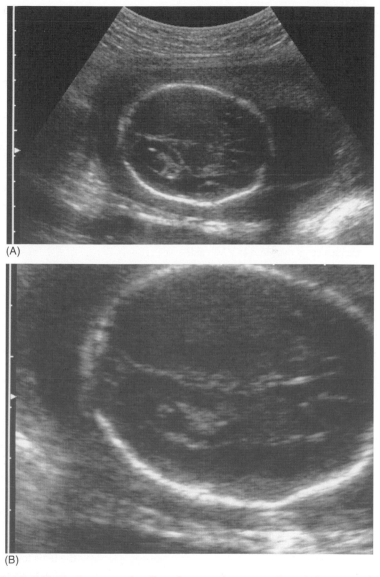

(A)

(B)

Fig. 1.4 (A,B) *Scenario – the effect of zoom to focus on a choroid plexus cyst. The focal zone is marked on screen with the small arrow on the left of each image.*

6. I wish to do some measurements.

Identify the *freeze* button. Each machine has its own menu options with calipers to measure distance or circumference. Obstetric tables are entered by the manufacturer according to your department's wishes and it is usually quite simple (after someone has shown you!) to bring these onto the side of the screen.

7. Anything else?

Yes, you need to be able to *print* off a frozen image and take a *video* recording. A useful facility to obtain your best image is the cineloop which replays the last few frames before the frozen image. All suspected abnormal findings should have a hard copy taken and suspected fetal abnormalities should be video recorded. Make sure the patient's initials and identity number are recorded also.

Finally, clean the coupling gel off the probe and lead. If you drop the probe on the floor, you could face a bill of £5000 for a replacement. Look after the equipment which costs the same as a Mercedes.

Checklist Machine controls – the basics

Choose probe	Freeze
Depth	Measure
Zoom	Obstetric tables
Gain	Print, video
Focal zone	

Artefact may occur in your image due to equipment problems, tissue effects and poor technique.

Equipment

Older equipment understandably will give poorer image quality. Adjustment of the gain, time gain compensation and focal zone may improve the image for you. Regular checks of the equipment should be undertaken, particularly for caliper measurements.

Tissue effects

These occur due to the type of tissue (e.g. bone causing shadowing, excessive abdominal wall fat causing weakening of the transmission pulses) or the interface between tissues (e.g. enhancement due to the ultrasound beam not being attenuated as it passes through fluid causing brightness distal to the fluid). Other types of recognised artefact are reverberation, mirror, comet effect, split image and slice thickness. Your image quality can be improved by scanning from a different angle and adjusting the overall gain and time gain compensation.

Many of the imaging artefacts occur in obese patients due to weakening of the transmission pulses. A feature to be found in recent ultrasound machines is tissue harmonic imaging. This reduces artefact and gives improved lateral resolution in deeper structures further from the probe.

Operator technique

If you are fortunate to have a choice of transducer, you may choose the wrong one resulting in the focal zone and frequency being set on the superficial structures. Noise on the screen will result if your gain is too high and banding will occur with the wrong time gain compensation settings. Finally, too much pressure can distort the image and, in addition, cause discomfort for the patient.

Safety

High levels of ultrasound cause heating, cavitation and streaming of fluid. Diagnostic ultrasound has been used for several decades now with no proven deleterious effects to the developing embryo. With the introduction of new techniques, continual vigilance is required. You should be aware that pulsed Doppler at maximum machine outputs and colour flow imaging with small colour boxes have the greatest potential for biological effects. Therefore, careful control of output levels and exposure times is required when using pulsed or colour Doppler. Routine examination with Doppler ultrasound of the first trimester embryo is considered inadvisable. As the fetus develops, and bone becomes mineralised, the possibility of heating increases and this should be remembered when examining the head and brain.

It is only relatively recently that manufacturers have had to display safety indices on-screen to assist in the monitoring of acoustic outputs. These are the thermal index (TI) and mechanical index (MI). You should monitor the TI and MI on screen and avoid unnecessary high values and prolonged exposure times. The TI should be less than 0.3 and the MI less than 0.5. In obstetric scans, the soft tissue thermal index (TIS) should be monitored in the first 8 weeks and the bone thermal index (TIB) thereafter. (Further information is available on www.efsumb.org.)

Ergonomics

The physical relationship between you and your ultrasound machine (the ergonomics) is important. If you adopt a good posture and position, your risk of repetitive strain injury will be significantly reduced. Your scanning stool and table should have the facility to adjust height. Manufacturers have improved the equipment and it is best if your legs can be placed on a foot rest under the control panel so that it is easily accessible to you without stretching. Position your joints as near neutral as possible. This means that you should avoid hyperextension or hyperflexion. Keep your spine straight. In our department we sit on the left hand side of the patient, using the right arm so that both operator and patient see the same monitor. There are other conventions but the important issue is that you are sitting comfortably (Fig. 1.5).

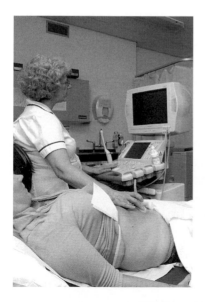
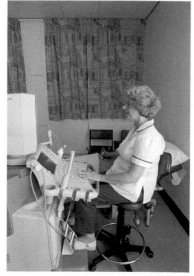

Fig. 1.5 Sonographer scanning comfortably.

Your training schedule

Acquiring the basic skill of ultrasound scanning requires the ability to visualise the two-dimensional image as a three-dimensional structure and to develop hand–eye coordination. Some people find this impossible and should not persevere to master the skill. Different levels of skill are acquired with time (Box 1.1), depending on the ultrasound investigation and caseload mix, but supervision is essential to avoid blunders. Some individuals acquire competence more quickly than others and your supervisor will decide when you are competent to report independently. You should plan your schedule as follows:

First level

You should undertake a weekly session for a minimum of 2 months acquiring at least 30 hours' supervised scanning. By this time you should expect to be competent to:

1. confirm intrauterine pregnancy

2. confirm viability

3. determine fetal number

4. undertake fetal measurements to determine gestational age and assess growth

5. determine presentation

6. assess liquor volume

7. note placental site

8. suspect abnormalities relating to the above and *seek a second opinion*.

Second level

With continued clinical ultrasound experience your competence will improve. When you have completed 100 sessions or 300 hours, you should expect to be competent to:

1. detect and specify early pregnancy complications

2. detect and specify fetal abnormalities

3. undertake assessment of the growth-restricted fetus

4. accurately locate the placental site

5. provide supervision and training.

Third level

Obstetricians developing subspecialty expertise in fetal medicine require to undertake training within a 3-year programme recognised by the Royal College of Obstetricians and Gynaecologists, at the end of which they should be clinically competent to:

1. receive regional referrals for difficult diagnosis

2. perform fetal interventions

3. provide regional training courses

4. have a commitment to research and development.

Box 1.1   Summary of levels of skills

Level 1 – 30 hours
Level 2 – 300 hours
Level 3 – 3 years

Log your cases

In addition to recording the time spent scanning, it is valuable to log your cases (Box 1.2) to assess the breadth of experience which you are gaining. There are many clinical indications to undertake an ultrasound examination but they can be broadly categorised as follows:

1. Early pregnancy (EP)

You should record the number of cases where the pregnancy is viable (10) or non-viable (10) and if there were any other findings – multiple (3), ectopic (1), intrauterine contraceptive device (IUCD) (1), fibroid (1), ovarian cyst (1). The numbers in brackets refer to the minimum experience you should have to acquire Level 1 expertise. At least five cases should be transvaginal (TV).

2. Detailed anomaly (DA)

After 30 cases, you should be able to recognise normality and deviations from this. Always get a second opinion when in doubt.

3. Late pregnancy assessment (LPA)

You should undertake at least 20 of these for Level 1 to acquire a basic level of competence to undertake fetal measurements, determine presentation, assess liquor volume and note placental site.

These three categories form the guide to your logbook and the following is an example of how you should put this into practice.

Box 1.2 **Example of logbook entries**				
Scan no.	Patient unit no.	Scan category (EP, DA, LPA)	Comment	Supervisor's signature
1	656453	EP	viable	
2	998976	EP	anembryonic (TV)	
3	556566	DA	normal	
4	556455	DA	choroid plexus cyst	
5	233342	LPA	normal growth	
6	888909	LPA	breech	

Reporting your findings

Your report should be standardised and structured according to the indication for the scan. This is dealt with in subsequent chapters.

Descriptive terms

You require to have a knowledge of different descriptive terms which you will need to describe your ultrasound images. These relate to the echo-density of the structures examined and range from echo-free (without internal echoes) to homogeneous (Box 1.3).

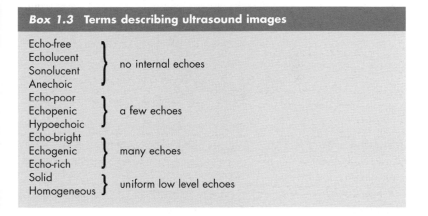

Box 1.3 Terms describing ultrasound images

Echo-free Echolucent Sonolucent Anechoic	no internal echoes
Echo-poor Echopenic Hypoechoic	a few echoes
Echo-bright Echogenic Echo-rich	many echoes
Solid Homogeneous	uniform low level echoes

Scanning planes

The median plane is the vertical anteroposterior one through the midline of the body and this plane and those parallel to it are termed the *sagittal* or *longitudinal* planes. At right angles to these are the *coronal* planes. These names are derived from the sagittal and coronal sutures of the skull. A horizontal section is usually referred to as the transverse plane (Fig. 1.6).

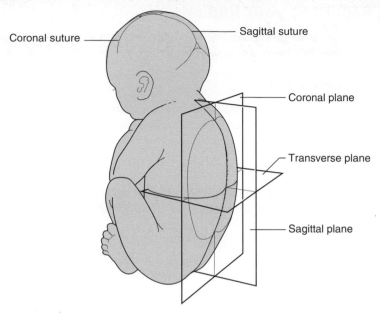

Coronal suture

Sagittal suture

Coronal plane

Transverse plane

Sagittal plane

Fig. 1.6 *Scanning planes.*

Early pregnancy

The viable pregnancy

The aims of early pregnancy scanning are to determine viability, gestational age and fetal number. In addition, the adnexa should be visualised to exclude significant pathology. Measurement of the crown–rump length (CRL) of the embryo in the first trimester has been shown to be the most accurate parameter for assessment of gestational age. This is because in the first trimester, there is little biological variation seen in the measurement taken in different patients at the same gestation and the percentage increase in size in a week is greatest at this time. Simple measurements to recall are:

CRL = 10 mm = mean for 7 weeks

CRL = 30 mm = mean for 9 weeks and 5 days

CRL = 60 mm = mean for 12 weeks and 3 days.

The measurements increase markedly in a short space of time (Figs 2.1–2.3).

1. *Calculate the gestational age* from the last menstrual period (LMP) before starting your scan so that you have an idea of what you expect to visualise. Always have ready access to a gestation wheel calculator. Gestational age is always based on completed weeks from the first day of the LMP. In a patient

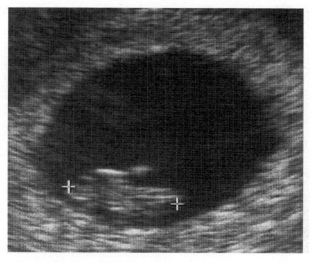

Fig. 2.1   *CRL 14 mm = 7w 4d.*

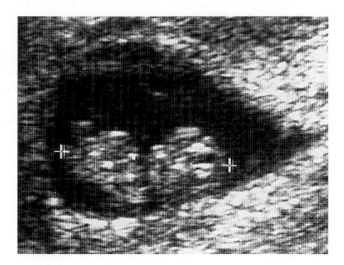

Fig. 2.2 *CRL 24 mm = 8w 6d.*

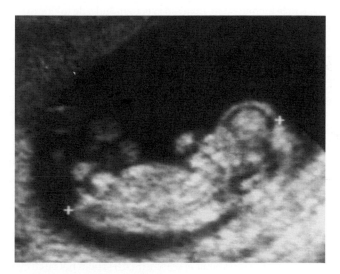

Fig. 2.3 *CRL 40 mm = 10w 5d.*

with a normal 28-day menstrual cycle, ovulation occurs on day 14 and conception very soon thereafter. Embryonic age therefore tends to be 2 weeks less than gestational age. A pill-withdrawal period can delay ovulation and a long menstrual cycle may make the true gestational age less than expected.

2. The patient should have a full bladder to aid *identification of the uterus*, especially before 10 weeks when the uterus is still well within the pelvis. If the bladder is empty, a transvaginal scan will be required unless the patient is very thin. The uterus is difficult to identify in the obese patient or when it is in a retroverted position. If you cannot define the uterine cavity transabdominally, a transvaginal scan will reveal all.

3. Identify an intrauterine gestation sac with a fetal pole and a fetal heart (FH) pulsation. Viability is confirmed when the *heart pulsation* is seen. Using transvaginal ultrasound, the gestation sac (Fig. 2.4) is first seen at 4.5 weeks and measures 2–4 mm. The earliest time at which the heart pulsation can be seen is 5 weeks when the embryonic length is 2–4 mm, but in 10% of viable pregnancies a pulsation will still not be visible. The circular yolk sac (Fig. 2.5) appears at 5 weeks as a 10 mm sac. It has no predictive value but confirms that the pregnancy is intrauterine. Using transabdominal ultrasound, the sequence of events is 1 week later.

4. Scan the whole uterine cavity from top to bottom and side to side to make sure there is only one fetus and that the outline of the sac appears smooth. You will miss a *multiple pregnancy* if you omit this step. At this step, you should look at the uterine wall to exclude fibroids, uterine abnormality and also look at the *adnexa* to exclude ovarian cysts.

5. Move the probe to obtain the longest image of the fetus, freeze the frame and measure the length from end to end. This is termed the *crown–rump length*. Repeat until you are satisfied that your measurements are consistent. Three times should be enough. Your machine will normally be programmed to convert this measurement to a gestational age. Be careful not to include the yolk sac which may be mistaken for the fetal head at early gestations. Late in the first trimester the measurement is less accurate because of fetal flexion as the following example shows (Fig. 2.6A,B).

6. Finally, check the gestation converted from the CRL against that from the menstrual dates. The measurement has an accuracy equivalent to + or – 4 days so that the patient's *expected date of delivery* (EDD) should not be changed if the difference equates to a week or less.

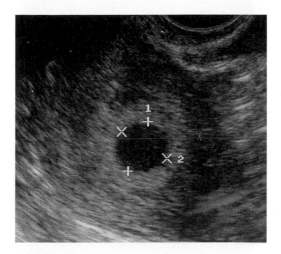

Fig. 2.4 *Intrauterine gestation sac at 4w 6d, measuring 12 × 11 mm.*

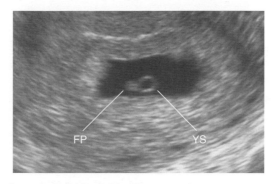

Fig. 2.5 *Yolk sac (YS) and fetal pole (FP) at 5w 3d.*

Case Scenario (Fig. 2.6A,B)

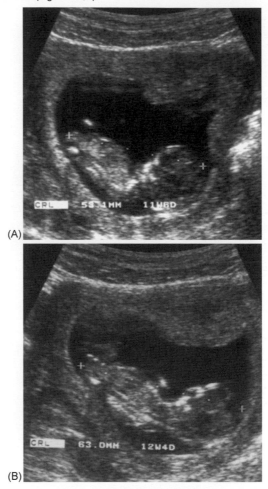

(A)

(B)

The above two measurements of the crown–rump length were taken on the same fetus. The patient had a gestational age of 12 weeks and 5 days by her certain LMP. The better, more accurate measurement equates to this gestation. It is important to obtain the longest measurement in the unflexed fetus.

Checklist

Calculate gestation from LMP
Identify the uterus and gestation sac
Look for FH pulsation to confirm viability
Exclude multiple pregnancy
Check adnexa
Measure CRL
Verify EDD

Points to remember

	Gestation of earliest ultrasound appearance	
	Transvaginal scan	Transabdominal scan
Intrauterine sac (2–4 mm)	4.5 weeks	5.5 weeks
FH pulsation, CRL 2–4 mm	5 weeks	6 weeks
Yolk sac (10 mm)	5 weeks	6 weeks

The non-viable pregnancy

When the FH pulsation is absent, the pregnancy is non-viable and will result in miscarriage. The patient may be asymptomatic or experience brown vaginal staining or frank bleeding. If there is no visible embryo and no FH, this is termed **anembryonic**. When the embryo can be measured and there is no FH, the diagnosis is that of **silent (delayed or missed) miscarriage**. Both findings are in keeping with early fetal demise. However, before considering a pregnancy non-viable, certain precautions are required and strict guidelines must be followed to avoid evacuation of an ongoing pregnancy.

A structured approach to your technique is required and a standardised report (see Box 2.1 on p. 30) should be given. You should be supervised until competent and, even then, a second opinion should be readily sought. The clinical history should be known to you and you should communicate your ultrasound scan findings to the patient. If the pregnancy is non-viable, counselling and emotional support will be required.

1. Know the *clinical history* before you start scanning. Bleeding in early pregnancy means that the patient is **threatening** to miscarry unless there is a local cause for the bleeding, such as a cervical polyp. If pain occurs, this may be due to uterine contractions trying to expel a blood clot or the conceptus. If cervical dilatation occurs then miscarriage becomes **inevitable**. If tissue is passed, miscarriage has occurred which is either incomplete or complete. Irregular echo-bright areas within the uterine cavity suggest that the miscarriage is **incomplete** (Fig. 2.7) but it is often not possible to differentiate blood clot from retained tissue. When all the products of conception have been passed and the cavity of the uterus is seen to be empty with a clear midline echo, then the miscarriage is **complete**.

2. When you experience difficulty visualising the fetal pole or FH transabdominally, undertake a *transvaginal scan* (see Ch. 7). The potential problems of a retroverted uterus and obesity causing poor resolution are immediately overcome and viability can be more easily ascertained once the uterine cavity is found. If the patient's bladder has been overfull, then she will be more comfortable after passing some urine. A little urine in the bladder is helpful for orientation.

3. Identify the *gestation sac*, check that it looks regular in outline, and that there is only one. It may appear irregular and collapsing or there may be evidence of haematoma formation (Fig. 2.8). There may be more than one sac so scan the uterus across its full breadth. Measure the diameters in three dimensions

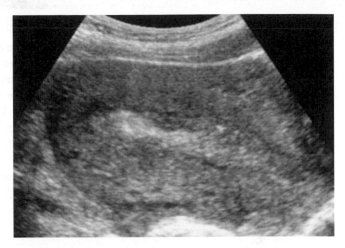

Fig. 2.7 *Echo-bright tissue seen within uterine cavity in keeping with an incomplete miscarriage.*

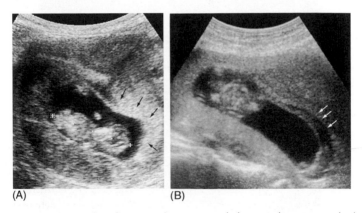

(A)   (B)

Fig. 2.8 *Two examples of retromembranous or subchorionic haematoma, both extending from the edge of the chorion frondosum (see Fig. 4.3 for embryology). In* **(A)** *the haematoma is echo-dense, suggestive of clot; in* **(B)** *it is echo-free.*

and take the average. If the mean diameter is more than 20 mm and there is no evidence of an embryo or yolk sac, the appearances are highly suggestive of an anembryonic pregnancy (Fig. 2.9). It is wise to obtain a second opinion

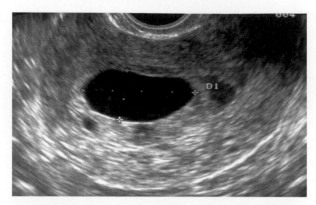

Fig. 2.9 (A) *Transvaginal scan showing empty gestation sac measuring 37 × 18 × 25 mm, highly suggestive of an anembryonic pregnancy.*

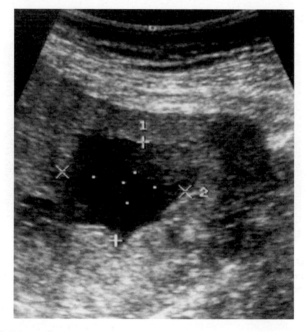

Fig. 2.9 (B) *Collapsing gestation sac measuring 25 × 27 × 28 mm in keeping with an anembryonic pregnancy.*

to confirm your findings. It is recommended to repeat the scan 7 days later for absolute confirmation unless clinical circumstances dictate otherwise.

4. Check the *contents* of the gestation sac and ascertain the presence or not of the yolk sac, FH and embryo. If the embryo is seen, measure the CRL. If this is greater than 6 mm with no evidence of an FH, the appearances are highly suggestive of a silent miscarriage (Fig. 2.10). Inform the patient and repeat the scan 7 days later for confirmation unless the clinical details suggest otherwise.

5. Consider the *differential diagnosis*. If you see a gestation sac, no fetal pole or FH, then you are dealing with either an early viable pregnancy, an anembryonic pregnancy or an ectopic pregnancy. The presence of a fetal pole, FH or yolk sac excludes an ectopic. If the mean sac diameter is less than 20 mm or the CRL less than 6 mm, a repeat scan should be undertaken to assess viability after at least 7 days. The scan is an investigation requested by the clinician who will consider all the clinical features of the case and make the final diagnosis.

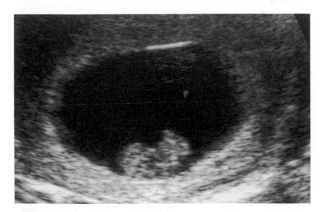

Fig. 2.10 *CRL 15 mm = 7w 5d. Fetus located at base of gestation sac. No fetal heart pulsation seen. The findings were in keeping with a silent miscarriage in this patient who was 12 weeks' pregnant and had experienced brown staining for 5 days.*

Descriptive terms for types of miscarriage

Threatened
Silent (delayed or missed)
Inevitable
Incomplete
Complete

Box 2.1 Example of a structured report

Date		
Type of scan	transabdominal	transvaginal
Gestation sac	yes	no
	regular	irregular
Mean sac diameter		
Fetal pole	yes	no
CRL		
Fetal heart pulsation	yes	no
Yolk sac	yes	no
Retained products	yes	no
Adnexal abnormality	yes	no
Free fluid in pelvis	yes	no
Comments		
Sonographer		

Checklist

Know clinical history
Do transvaginal scan
Identify gestation sac – number, outline, haematoma
Evaluate contents – yolk sac, FH, embryo
Consider differential diagnosis – wrong dates, non-viable, ectopic
Communicate with patient
Issue structured report

Points to remember

1. A mean diameter more than 20 mm with no evidence of an embryo or yolk sac is highly suggestive of an anembryonic pregnancy.
2. A CRL greater than 6 mm with no evidence of an FH is highly suggestive of a silent miscarriage.
3. A repeat transvaginal scan 7 days later should confirm the diagnosis.

Case Scenario (Fig. 2.11A,B)

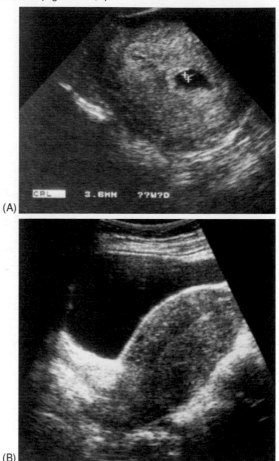

(A)

(B)

*The patient presented with vaginal bleeding at 6 weeks' gestation and the first scan **(A)** showed an intrauterine sac measuring 17 × 23 mm. There was a small fetal pole measuring 3.6 mm with no fetal heart pulsation. The measurements were less than those required to make a firm diagnosis of early fetal demise and the patient was asked to return in 1 week. She had passed tissue and the scan **(B)** revealed an empty uterus with a clear midline echo in keeping with complete miscarriage.*

Case Scenario (Fig. 2.12A–C)

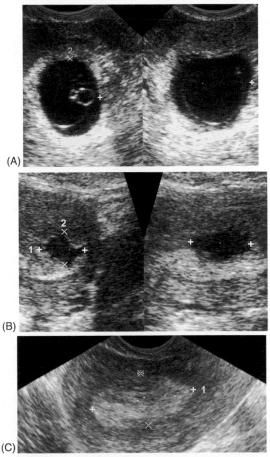

(A)

(B)

(C)

*The patient presented at 6 weeks' gestation with vaginal bleeding. **(A)** Yolk sac and adjacent small fetal pole were seen. There was a fetal heart pulsation and so the pregnancy was considered viable. The patient continued bleeding and **(B)** was taken 1 week later. This revealed a collapsing gestation sac, with mean diameter of 15 mm. There was no fetal pulsation or pole identifiable. The patient was informed of the findings and wished conservative management. She returned 10 days later with heavy bleeding and gave a history of having passed tissue. A repeat scan **(C)** revealed that the uterine cavity contained an echo-bright area measuring 36 × 18 mm in keeping with retained products. The patient opted for a surgical evacuation of retained products.*

Ectopic pregnancy

The classic symptoms of ectopic pregnancy are secondary amenorrhoea, vaginal bleeding and abdominal pain but any combination is possible. Your ultrasound findings will not always be conclusive and are more likely to be only suggestive of ectopic pregnancy. Your report will aid the diagnosis in association with the symptoms, signs and serum human chorionic gonadotrophin (hCG) levels. A transvaginal scan is usually necessary.

1. Your suspicions should be aroused when you have difficulty identifying a viable intrauterine pregnancy. If the *uterine cavity* appears empty and the patient has a definite positive pregnancy test, an ectopic pregnancy is highly likely unless the history is suggestive of complete miscarriage. However, the intrauterine appearances may be less clear because of the hormonal influences of pregnancy causing the endometrium to decidualise such that a pseudodecidual or pseudogestational sac becomes evident. This is present in around 15% of ectopic pregnancies. It contains endometrial fluid, is usually less than 10 mm, is centrally located within the uterine cavity and may be surrounded by a single echogenic rim. The normal chorionic sac is eccentrically placed within the uterine cavity. In practice, it is often difficult to differentiate a true intrauterine gestation sac (Fig. 2.4) from a pseudogestational sac (Figs 2.13–2.15), especially when the sac is less than

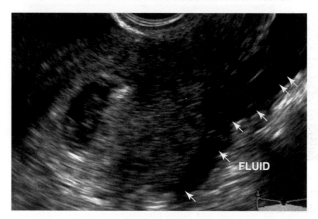

FLUID

Fig. 2.13 *Transvaginal scan showing pseudogestational sac within the uterus and significant fluid in the pouch of Douglas. This patient went on to have a laparotomy and right salpingectomy. Her haemoglobin was 7 g/dl and there was 1000 ml blood in the peritoneal cavity.*

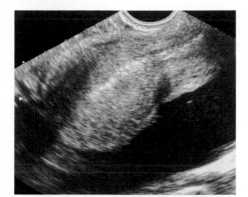

Fig. 2.14 *A case of ectopic pregnancy with empty uterus and fluid in the pouch of Douglas. This was found to be equivalent to 500 ml blood.*

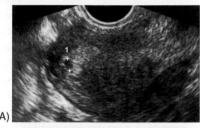

(A)

Fig. 2.15 (A,B) *Different appearances of 'intrauterine sac' in cases of ectopic pregnancy.*

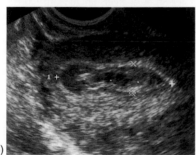

(B)

5 mm. Such decidualised endometrium may be passed by the patient sometimes as a decidual cast when it may look like products of conception.

2. Always look at the *adnexa*. Abnormalities are seen in 70% of ectopic pregnancies but the appearances are variable and frequently only suggestive and not diagnostic of an ectopic pregnancy. You can only be absolutely certain if an intact

gestation sac with a positive FH is seen outside the uterine cavity. You can be almost certain when you see in the adnexum near the ovary a hyperechoic ring around a gestation sac (the bagel or doughnut sign). The most common finding is a small non-cystic mass with mixed echoes next to the ovary. Haemorrhage around a sac and rupture of the fallopian tube explain the variations which are seen. The corpus luteum is found on the same side of the ectopic in 80% of cases. However, a corpus luteum, pelvic inflammatory disease, endometriosis, hydrosalpinges and small bowel can all give similar ultrasonic appearances to an ectopic.

3. Finally, evaluate the *pouch of Douglas* for free fluid. If the patient has had significant haemorrhage, an echo-free area is seen behind the uterus (Figs 2.13, 2.14). However, a small amount of free fluid can be a normal finding.

4. Consider the *differential diagnosis*. The patient may have an early viable or non-viable pregnancy. It may only be over the course of a week that the true diagnosis evolves. Your ultrasound findings will be interpreted in association with the serum hCG levels which greatly improve the diagnostic accuracy. When the serum levels are more than 1500 IU/l, an intrauterine sac will be seen in 90% of viable pregnancies using transvaginal ultrasound. However, the levels vary depending on the assay used and the experience of the sonographer. This discriminatory cut-off is higher for transabdominal scanning when the cut-off is 6500 IU/l. In a viable pregnancy, serum hCG levels range from 100 IU/l at the first missed period to 50–100 000 IU/l at 10 weeks, falling to 10–20 000 at 20 weeks and remain around that level until term. The levels double every 2 days at values below 1200 IU/l and every 3 days below 6000 IU/l. In an ectopic or non-viable pregnancy this will not happen.

Checklist

Know clinical features
Evaluate intrauterine appearances with transvaginal scan
Check adnexa and pouch of Douglas
Consider differential diagnosis – early viable, non-viable or ectopic

---

Points to remember

1. When the serum hCG is greater than 1000 IU/l, an intrauterine sac should be seen using a transvaginal probe.
2. hCG levels double every 2 days below 1200 IU/l and every 3 days below 6000 IU/l.
3. hCG levels reach a maximum of 50–100 000 IU/l at 10 weeks.

Case Scenario (Fig. 2.16)

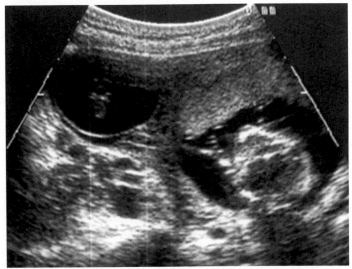

This image shows the rare occurrence of an intrauterine and a co-existing cornual ectopic pregnancy. The patient had a laparotomy at 18 weeks' gestation because of persisting abdominal pain. The ectopic was removed and the uterine wall sutured. The patient went on to have an elective caesarean section at 38 weeks. This is known as a heterotopic pregnancy, where there are co-existing intrauterine and extrauterine gestations. The risk of this occurring spontaneously is 1 in 10–50 000 but it is much higher in assisted conceptions, around 1 in 4000.

2.4

Multiple pregnancy

A first-trimester scan is essential for the reliable identification of chorionicity and amnionicity in multiple pregnancy. Perinatal mortality is higher in monochorionic twin pregnancies because of the sharing of a common circulation and in monoamniotic ones because of the sharing of one sac. An understanding of the embryological formation of a twin pregnancy is required to aid interpretation of your scan findings.

Embryology

In a dizygotic twin pregnancy, two eggs are fertilised and implant separately, resulting in non-identical twins. Thus, each embryo has its own gestational or chorionic sac and the pregnancy is always dichorionic, diamniotic (Fig. 2.17). In a monozygotic twin pregnancy, one egg is fertilised and the zygote divides later, resulting in identical twins. Thirty per cent of fertilised eggs will divide before implantation and result in a dichorionic, diamniotic pregnancy; the remaining 70% divide after implantation and all are monochorionic (Box 2.2). The amnionicity depends on when the division occurs after implantation: 4–8 days afterwards results in a diamniotic twin pregnancy, 8–13 days in a monoamniotic twin pregnancy and 13–16 days in a monoamniotic but conjoined twin pregnancy. Therefore, the later the division of the zygote, the more problematic the outcome is likely to be.

1. Your *detection* of a twin pregnancy is usually unexpected, but more common following assisted reproduction. The patient is not always happy with the news. You must visualise two embryos on the screen at the same time. The viability of each embryo must be confirmed with identification of a positive FH. Always check that you have not missed other embryos by scanning the whole uterine cavity transversely and longitudinally. Undertake a transvaginal scan to establish chorionicity and amnionicity.

2. You can establish the *chorionicity* as early as 5 weeks' gestation by simply seeing the number of sacs. Undercounting may occur at this time and a repeat scan should be booked at 9–14 weeks' gestation.

3. You can establish *amnionicity* at 8 weeks when the amnion is seen separately from the embryo. The extra-amniotic space diminishes as the amniotic sac grows and the chorion and amnion fuse. In a dichorionic, diamniotic twin

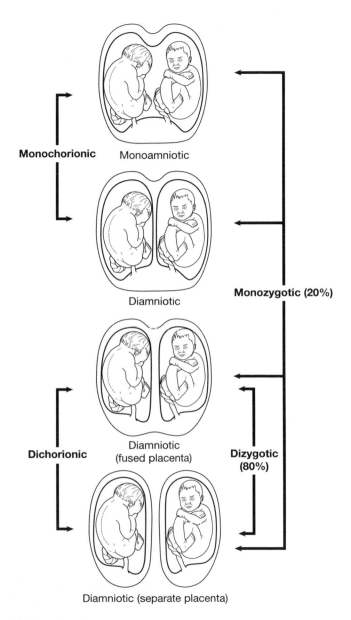

Monochorionic Monoamniotic

Diamniotic

Monozygotic (20%)

Dichorionic Diamniotic
(fused placenta)

**Dizygotic
(80%)**

Diamniotic (separate placenta)

Fig. 2.17 *Embryology of a twin pregnancy.*

Points to remember

1. Dichorionic, diamniotic pregnancies have the lowest perinatal mortality.
2. The lambda sign is seen in dichorionic twin pregnancies.
3. The dividing membrane is thin and at right angles to the uterine wall in monochorionic diamniotic twin pregnancies.
4. In a dichorionic pregnancy, the twins may be monozygotic or dizygotic.
5. In a monochorionic pregnancy, the twins are always monozygotic (identical).
6. By 20 weeks, about 10% of dichorionic pregnancies will not have a lambda sign. Measurement of membrane thickness and determination of fetal gender and number of placentae may help.

Molar pregnancy

Complete (or hydatidiform) mole is a rare event in pregnancy in the UK (1 in 3000) but is more common in the Far East (1 in 300). It is associated with the clinical features of vaginal bleeding, hyperemesis, hypertension and large for dates. There is a subsequent 10–20% risk of choriocarcinoma and registration of all molar pregnancies is essential so that reliable follow-up of urinary hCG levels can be undertaken. The karyotype is typically diploid (46XX) in 95% of cases and this is of paternal origin.

Ultrasound is not reliable in making the diagnosis of partial mole in the first trimester and histological confirmation of abnormal trophoblastic proliferation is required. Ninety per cent of partial moles are triploid (69XXX or 69XXY) and if they survive the first trimester, early intrauterine growth restriction (IUGR) will become apparent from 16 weeks. The subsequent risk of malignancy after a partial mole is 0.5–3% and registration of the pregnancy loss with a regional centre for hCG follow-up must be ensured.

1. You will not have difficulty making the diagnosis of a *hydatidiform mole*. You may detect this at a routine, early pregnancy scan or the patient may be referred with bleeding which is a very common presentation. When you scan the uterus, it will be full of multiple sonolucent spaces which are the small grape-like vesicles of the mole (Fig. 2.22). There is no embryonic tissue. In 20%, theca lutein cysts are also found. Rarely, a twin pregnancy may be found where there is a complete mole and a viable co-twin.

2. You may find ultrasonic features which are suggestive of *partial molar change*. In the first trimester, these are seen typically in a silent miscarriage when the fetus may have been dead for some time and hydropic change has occurred in the chorion. You will find multiple echo-free areas within the chorion and sometimes within the amniotic cavity. These represent hydropic change and histology is necessary to verify the diagnosis. In the second trimester, the placenta will appear enlarged with multicystic, avascular, sonolucent areas. At the time of a detailed scan at 18–22 weeks, the placenta will be obviously enlarged (>4 cm) and early IUGR will be apparent.

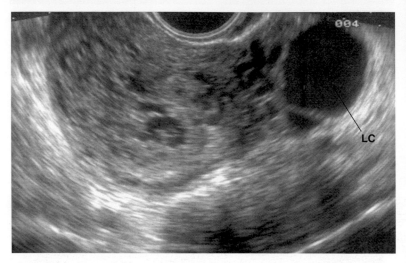

Fig. 2.22 *Multiple echo-free cysts seen within the uterine cavity in keeping with a hydatidiform mole. There is also a luteal cyst (LC) measuring 3 cm in diameter.*

Case Scenario (Fig. 2.23)

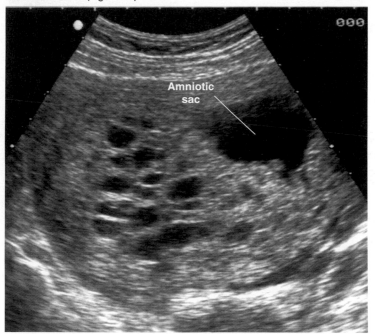

Amniotic
sac

This scan shows hydropic change within the chorion. There was also a fetus in the amniotic sac (not seen in print) with CRL 63 mm = 12w 4d. The patient at the time of the scan was 20 weeks' pregnant and had had an early pregnancy scan at 9 weeks confirming viability and gestation. It appeared that a silent miscarriage had occurred with degenerative changes in the chorion. The pregnancy was terminated and histology of the chorion revealed partial molar change. The karyotype was found to be triploidy (69XXY). The patient was registered for serial hCG follow-up.

Points to remember

1. A complete mole can be diagnosed by ultrasound in the first trimester.
2. A partial mole may be suspected on ultrasound in the second trimester and is associated with triploidy in 90% of cases.
3. All partial and complete moles must be registered for urinary hCG follow-up.

Nuchal translucency

Nuchal translucency (NT) measurement assesses the lymphatic fluid which accumulates under the skin at the back of the fetal neck. The measurement is undertaken between 10 and 14 weeks (CRL between 45 and 84 mm) when the lymphatic system is developing. It is easiest to do at 12 weeks. High-resolution equipment is required and the acquisition of a correct measurement may take up to 15 minutes and requires patience.

There is a 10% risk of major abnormality when the measurement is more than 3 mm, increasing to 90% at more than 6 mm. The abnormalities are mainly chromosomal and, to a lesser extent, cardiac and neuromuscular. It follows that if the karyotype is normal when the measurement is increased, further detailed scans should be done.

The actual risk for trisomy 21 can be calculated, incorporating maternal age and measurement of NT, CRL, serum free β-human chorionic gonadotrophin and pregnancy associated plasma protein-A (PAPP-A).

1. Inform the patient that this is a *screening test* in which an abnormal measurement could be found that may be associated with an abnormality and so further tests may be required. A normal measurement does not guarantee normality. Make sure the patient wishes to have the test.

2. Identify the longitudinal axis of the fetus as you would for a CRL measurement and obtain a *sagittal view* of the fetus visualising the length of the spine. The fetus should be in the neutral position and not hyperextended.

3. Identify the *amnion* separately from the skin at the back of the neck. When fetal movement occurs, the two can usually be distinguished. This is essential otherwise you may overestimate the true measurement.

4. Magnify the image to visualise the fetal head and upper thorax. Reduce the gain to sharpen the edges for caliper placement. Tissue harmonic imaging falsely thickens the lines and should not be used.

5. Identify the echo-free area at the back of the neck and measure the maximum *translucent distance* between the skin and soft tissues overlying the cervical spine (Fig. 2.24). Repeat until you are satisfied and take the maximum measurement (Figs 2.25, 2.26).

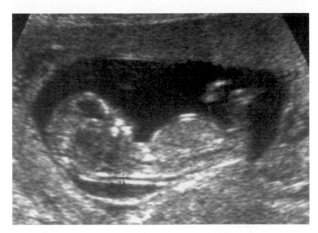

Fig. 2.24 *Measurement of nuchal translucency. Note that the amnion is seen separately.*

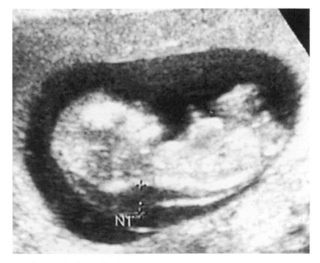

Fig. 2.25 *The nuchal translucency measurement was 6.2 mm.*

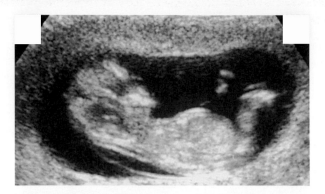

Fig. 2.26 *Is the nuchal translucency measurement increased or not? It was normal. A falsely enlarged measurement could easily be made if the amnion was incorporated. Be careful to avoid this mistake.*

Checklist

Counsel the patient
Obtain a sagittal view of the fetus in the neutral position
Visualise amnion as a separate entity
Magnify, reduce gain, avoid harmonic imaging
Measure maximum nuchal translucency
Take print and check for image size, head position, amnion, skin line and caliper placement

---

Points to remember

1. Increased nuchal translucency (>3 mm) is associated with chromosomal and other abnormalities.
2. The measurement is made at 10–14 weeks (CRL 45–84 mm).
3. Always identify the amnion separately to avoid a false-positive.

Fetal abnormalities

Early pregnancy scanning at 11–14 weeks can detect certain fetal abnormalities. Detection rates are better after 13 weeks and improved with the use of transvaginal scanning. However, caution is required and you should be aware of the potential pitfalls which are related to embryological development.

1. The lateral ventricles occupy most of the cerebral hemispheres and within each the choroid plexus is very prominent. This is not hydrocephalus. Before this, at 7–9 weeks, the forebrain appears as a single ventricle.

2. Midgut herniation into the umbilical cord is physiological between 8 and 12 weeks (Fig. 2.27). This should not be mistaken for exomphalos which is more likely when the mean diameter of the herniated sac exceeds 7 mm and the CRL is more than 68 mm.

3. Renal function begins at 11 weeks and amniotic fluid volume may be normal in the first trimester, even with renal agenesis.

Detailed anatomical screening in early pregnancy is not standard practice and is restricted to patients at high risk of anomaly. However, you should be aware of certain gross structural abnormalities which are easily identified in the first trimester and which you will encounter in routine practice.

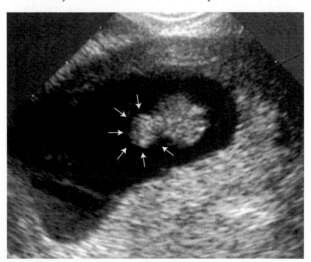

Fig. 2.27 *Physiological midgut herniation seen at 10 weeks. A repeat scan 3 weeks later revealed an intact abdominal wall.*

49

Anencephaly

This is absence of the cranium of the skull and brain. Skull ossification begins at 10 weeks and is complete by 12 weeks so it is normally after this time that the diagnosis is made.

At this early gestation brain tissue may be seen. Thus, the profile of the head may appear normal or have a herniated appearance with brain seemingly intact but no vault of skull. This is termed exencephaly (Fig. 2.28). This floating, exposed brain tissue lyses with advancing gestation.

1. In the sagittal view, you will suspect anencephaly when the top of the skull appears very small (Fig. 2.29).

2. Measure the CRL and this will be less than expected for the gestation.

3. Measure the femur length (FL) and this will correspond to the gestation.

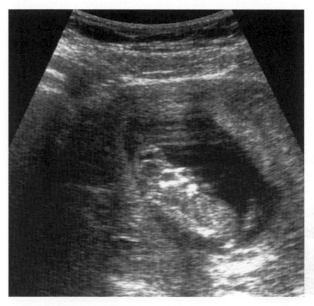

Fig. 2.28 *Exencephaly at 10 weeks.*

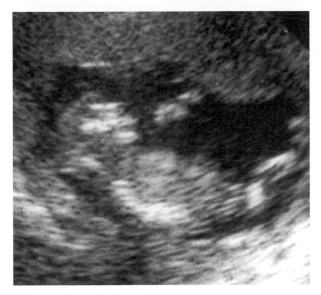

Fig. 2.29 *Anencephaly at 12 weeks.*

4. Now try to obtain a view of the face and the diagnosis will be obvious when you see a frog-like appearance (Fig. 2.30).

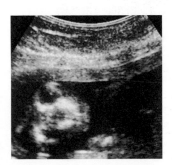

Fig. 2.30 *Same fetus as in Fig. 2.29 showing frog eye appearance.*

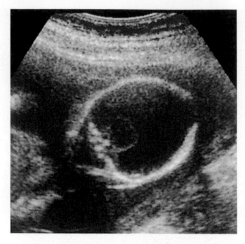

Fig. 2.31 *Holoprosencephaly seen at 14 weeks. The pregnancy was terminated.*

Holoprosencephaly

This occurs when there is incomplete division of the brain into cerebral hemispheres and lateral ventricles. The interhemispheric fissure, the lateral ventricles and the thalami may be partly or completely fused resulting in semilobar or lobar holoprosencephaly. This is a midline defect and there are usually associated facial abnormalities. The most severe forms are diagnosed at the end of the first trimester and have a strong association with trisomy 13 (Fig. 2.31).

1. You will suspect the diagnosis on a transverse view of the head at 12–14 weeks. Be careful that you do not falsely diagnose the condition because each lateral ventricle normally occupies most of the cerebral hemisphere but contains a prominent choroid plexus.

2. In the severe form, you will see a single ventricle with no midline echo. The thalami will be fused and protrude into the monoventricle. A rim of cerebral cortex will be evident.

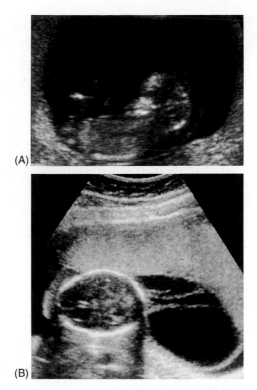

Fig. 2.32 *(A) Cystic hygroma. Chorion biopsy was undertaken and the karyotype was reported as 45XO (Turner's syndrome) and the parents opted not to continue with the pregnancy. (B) Septated cystic hygroma. This fetus was subsequently found to have trisomy 18.*

Cystic hygroma

Cystic hygromas are bilateral collections of lymphatic fluid which gather in the posterolateral region of the neck. They are classified as non-septated when the cystic spaces are seen on either side (Fig. 2.32A) and septated when the collection is more extensive around the back of the neck and divided by septa (Fig. 2.32B). There is probably a progression in severity from increased nuchal translucency in non-septated cystic hygroma to septated. Finally, generalised hydrops may be found (Fig. 2.33) and this carries a very poor prognosis. With cystic hygroma there is an

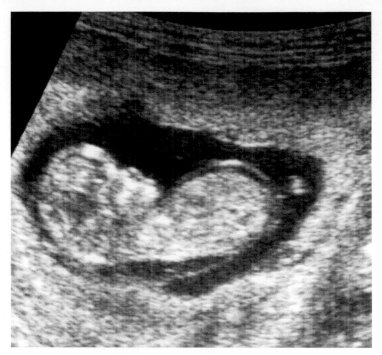

Fig. 2.33 *Generalised hydrops at 12 weeks. This patient opted not to have prenatal diagnosis and returned for a repeat scan at 15 weeks when no fetal heart pulsation was present. Chromosomal analysis of chorion taken after the miscarriage revealed 47XX+18 (trisomy 18).*

80% chance of chromosomal abnormality, mainly the trisomies and Turner's syndrome. If the pregnancy continues, hygromas become less obvious and tend to resolve.

1. You will suspect the diagnosis when you obtain a sagittal view of the fetus.

2. Confirm your diagnosis by viewing a transverse scan through the fetal neck and determine whether there are septations or not.

3. Check for evidence of hydrops.

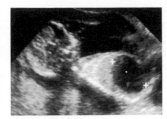

Fig. 2.34 *Distended bladder measuring 21 mm in diameter. Chorion biopsy revealed that this fetus had 47XY+18 (trisomy 18).*

Case Scenario (Fig. 2.35)

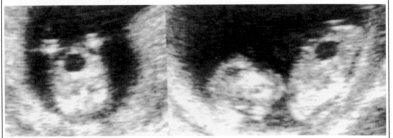

This 5 mm diameter intra-abdominal cystic structure was seen at 13 weeks gestation. At 16 weeks it was no longer present and the baby was normal at birth.

Points to remember

1. The lateral ventricles occupy most of the cerebral hemispheres.
2. The choroid plexus is very prominent.
3. Midgut herniation is physiological between 8 and 12 weeks.
4. There is little renal contribution to amniotic fluid in the first trimester.
5. Anencephaly, cystic hygroma, distended bladder and holoprosencephaly are the fetal abnormalities most commonly diagnosed in the first trimester.

4. The patient now will require counselling and the need for prenatal diagnosis which is normally chorion biopsy at this gestation.

Bladder outlet obstruction

Posterior urethral valves in male fetuses and urethral atresia in females result in a distended bladder which may be detected in the first trimester. There may be reduced or normal amniotic fluid; hydronephrosis is seen in about 50%. The upper limit of normal is 6 mm for the longitudinal diameter and more than 16 mm is associated with subsequent severe uropathy. There is a significant risk of chromosomal abnormality.

1. On sagittal section of the fetus you will see the distended bladder (Fig. 2.34).

2. Measure the longitudinal diameter.

3. Assess the amniotic fluid and look for hydronephrosis.

4. Counselling is required. This includes the option of termination, karyotyping and regular surveillance. A shunt may be necessary if oligohydramnios develops.

Associated findings

When you undertake an early pregnancy scan, you may find associated abnormalities within the uterine cavity, within the myometrium or outside the uterus in the adnexa.

Intrauterine

A. Uterine abnormality

This may be seen as a coincidental finding and you will see an empty cavity adjoining the pregnancy sac (Fig. 2.36). Unless it is already known, it is difficult ultrasonically to specify the exact type of uterine abnormality since the embryological variations are immense. Various types of uterine abnormality are described

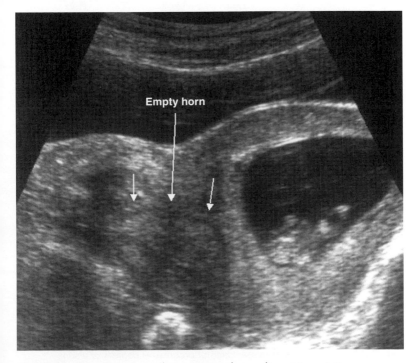

Fig. 2.36 *Bicornuate uterus showing empty horn adjacent to gestation sac.*

(Fig. 2.37); these are due to incomplete fusion of the two paramesonephric ducts in the embryo.

B. Intrauterine contraceptive device

A patient may have conceived with an IUCD in situ. You must identify whether it is within the uterus or not. It is important to describe its location because the obstetrician prefers to remove it to reduce the risk of miscarriage or infection. However, if the IUCD is at the fundus of the uterus, it would be unwise to attempt to remove it since the procedure itself is likely to cause miscarriage. Con-

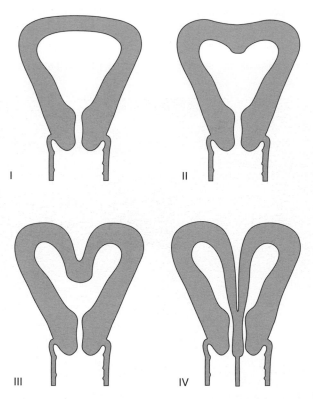

Fig. 2.37 *Diagrammatic representation of progressive degrees of uterine abnormality. I, normal; II arcuate; III bicornuate; IV double.*

versely, you may find that the IUCD is lying at the internal cervical os and it can then be simply removed. Sometimes it is outwith the uterine cavity and you will not see it ultrasonically. Such a patient will require an X-ray postpartum.

1. Look for the echogenic IUCD which appears as a rod-like structure. You require to scan the whole of the uterine contents from superior to inferior and left to right.

2. When you identify the IUCD, describe its location within the uterus and its relationship to the chorion, and whether it is embedded or not (Fig. 2.38).

Uterine

Within the wall of the uterus you may find one or more fibroids, benign growths of the uterine muscle. In pregnancy, they may enlarge and become more vascular but usually cause no problems. Occasionally, they outstrip their blood supply and undergo 'red degeneration' which is associated with pain.

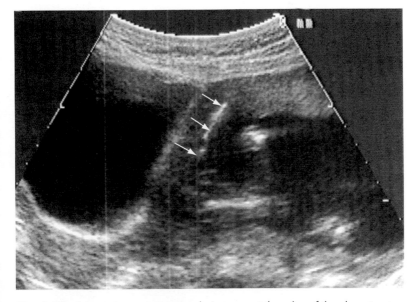

Fig. 2.38 *Intrauterine contraceptive device seen at the edge of the placenta at 16 weeks. The thread was not visible vaginally so it could not be removed. The pregnancy progressed without problems.*

59

1. Describe their location in the uterus and their size, giving a mean diameter. If large and near the cervix, they can obstruct descent of the head in labour. They may be submucosal, intramural or subserosal (Fig. 8.15). If submucosal or intramural, they may distort the uterine cavity. Usually this does not cause a problem but, rarely, may be associated with recurrent miscarriage or compression deformity of the fetus.

2. Describe their ultrasonic appearance. They normally appear homogeneous but they may have echo-bright areas in keeping with calcification or echo-free areas in keeping with degeneration.

Case Scenario (Fig. 2.39)

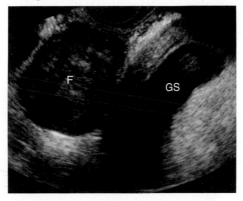

This patient was referred for a second opinion because of the finding of a suspected bicornuate uterus. However, this is an intramural fibroid (F). (GS = gestation sac.)

Case Scenario (Fig. 2.40)

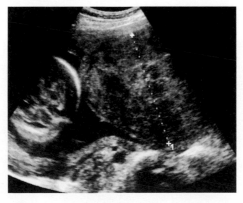

This fibroid, measuring 9.6 cm diameter, occupied the lower uterine segment preventing descent of the fetal head. The fetus was lying transversely and had to be delivered by classical (vertical incision in upper segment) caesarean section.

Extrauterine

You may detect an adnexal mass at the time of an early pregnancy scan. You require to consider the differential diagnosis (Box 2.3). The most common finding is an ovarian cyst. Most of these are unilocular and less than 6 cm (Fig. 2.41). These are physiological follicular cysts which have developed under the hormonal influences of pregnancy and require no action. Those larger than 6 cm may cause symptoms of pain if they undergo torsion or may obstruct labour. If the appearances are benign and the CA125 is normal, then the obstetrician may decide to manage conservatively and simply scan the patient 6 weeks postpartum. If the cyst is multiloculated or contains solid components, then this is of more concern and the possibility of malignancy cannot be ruled out. These are usually surgically removed.

Box 2.3 Differential diagnosis of adnexal mass

Ovarian cyst	Bladder diverticulum
Fibroid	Pelvic kidney
Hydrosalpinx	Retroperitoneal neoplasm
Dilated bowel	Heterotopic pregnancy

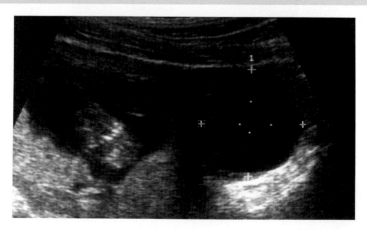

Fig. 2.41 *34 × 32 mm left echo-free unilocular ovarian cyst containing no solid components. The gestational age was 12 weeks. This was physiological and resolved spontaneously.*

Case Scenario (Fig. 2.42)

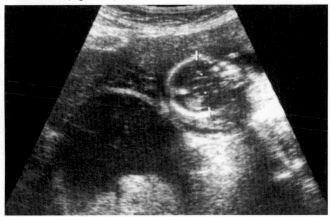

This 8 cm ovarian cyst was visualised at 14 weeks' gestation in a 19-year-old primigravid. It contained solid areas. The findings were suggestive of a dermoid (benign teratoma) cyst. A left oophorectomy was performed and the histology confirmed a benign teratoma.

Case Scenario (Fig. 2.43)

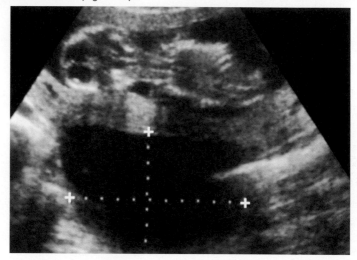

This unilocular 6.2 × 7.2 cm ovarian cyst lying in the pouch of Douglas was seen at 15 weeks' gestation. There were no solid components. The patient was asymptomatic. She was informed of the benign appearances and small risk of torsion. Conservative management was adopted and the patient had a follow-up scan 6 weeks after delivery. The cyst had resolved spontaneously.

Describe the position of the cyst, its size, whether it is unilocular or multilocular and whether there are solid components or not.

When you detect an adnexal mass, describe:

1. The position in relationship to the uterus.

2. The size in two dimensions which is usually sufficient.

3. The ultrasonic appearance, whether unilocular or multilocular, whether echo-free or with solid components.

Checklist

Uterine abnormality – adjoining empty cavity
IUCD – scan entire uterine contents to locate, describe in relation to uterine cavity and chorion
Fibroids – position, size, appearance
Ovarian cyst – position, size, appearance, locules, solid components
Adnexal mass – consider differential diagnosis

Points to remember

1. If you visualise an IUCD within the uterine cavity, describe its exact location and relationship to the chorion.
2. If fibroids are present, count them, describe their location and whether or not they distort the uterine cavity.
3. Unilocular ovarian cysts less than 6 cm are usually physiological.

The detailed anomaly scan

You will normally undertake this examination between 18 and 22 weeks when the structures can be visualised most clearly. The ability to assess normality is essential before you will be able to detect abnormality. A routine and systematic approach is necessary and you should issue a systematic report confirming the structures you have visualised. Some structures may not be clearly seen owing to maternal obesity or fetal position.

Before you begin your detailed scan, it is important to inform the patient what you are about to do. State that you are about to undertake a detailed scan to look at the structures in the fetus and that you may pick up a problem. Emphasise that not all problems are detected by ultrasound scanning and that the detailed scan is never a guarantee of normality. Ideally the patient will have had an information sheet giving details of your departmental policy on the anomaly scan and what structures are visualised.

If you suspect a problem, convey this finding to the patient and obtain a second opinion. Hard copies and video recordings should be made. Remember to complete your full structural survey and check for additional abnormalities. Onward referral to a fetal medicine specialist may be required for further assessment and karyotyping.

The head

Ultrasonic assessment of the head entails confirmation of the integrity of the skull bones, visualisation of the internal structures of the brain, assessment of the orbits, lips and, if time permits, the facial profile and ears. The following description of the fetal brain should be read in conjunction with Figures 3.1–3.4.

Anatomy of the brain

The forebrain is the location of the two cerebral hemispheres and the thalamus. Within each is the lateral ventricle which contains the choroid plexus and these vascular echogenic structures produce most of the cerebrospinal fluid (CSF). This flows through the interventricular foramina (of Monro) to the third and fourth ventricles and then escapes into the subarachnoid space. The central third ventricle is very narrow because of the development of the thalamus on either side. The roof of the third ventricle is formed by the corpus callosum which is a mass of white fibres connecting each hemisphere. The corpus callosum also spreads

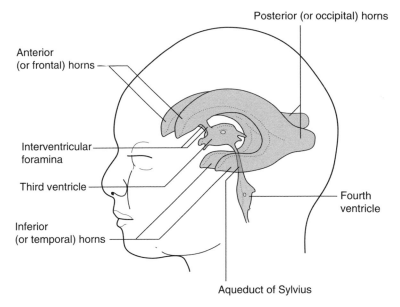

Fig. 3.1 *The cerebral ventricles.*

anteriorly to roof the lateral ventricle. The growth of the corpus callosum results in the lateral ventricles being separated by a thin partition, the septum pellucidum, which develops a median space called the cavum. This has no connection with the ventricles.

The midbrain contains the narrow aqueduct (of Silvius) and connects the third to the fourth ventricle in the hindbrain which lies anterior to the cerebellum, or little brain, in the posterior fossa of the skull.

Visualisation of the brain

There are three standard planes which you should be familiar with to view the fetal brain structures at 18–20 weeks (Fig. 3.2):

A. The transthalamic (Fig. 3.3)

This plane is obtained to measure the biparietal diameter (BPD) and thus ascertain gestational age between 13 and 22 weeks with an accuracy of 5–10 days. After that time the biological variation becomes too great and the measurement can mislead by up to 4 weeks after 30 weeks.

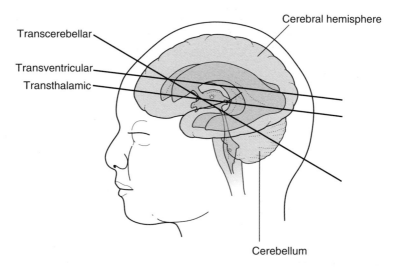

Fig. 3.2 *The three standard planes.*

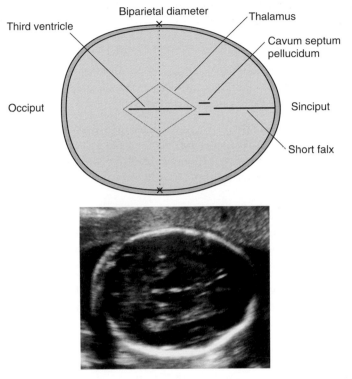

Fig. 3.3 *The transthalamic plane.*

1. Obtain an *oval* transverse section of the head. Look at the outline carefully. A lemon shape may be seen in association with spina bifida when each frontal bone appears concave. A posterior bony defect with herniation of the brain is pathognomonic of encephalocele.

2. Move the probe to view the *thalamic nuclei* which are easy to identify as sonolucent triangles on either side of the midline. They are separated by the third ventricle which is very thin.

3. Between the thalami and the sinciput, look for the short midline echo which constitutes the falx cerebri, a dense band of fibrous tissue separating the frontal lobes at this level. A long midline echo means you are too close to the vault.

4. Identify the rectangular echo-free *cavum septum pellucidum* between the falx and the third ventricle.

5. You can also visualise the *frontal* and *occipital horns* which are seen in this plane.

6. Measure the *BPD* from the upper edge of the proximal parietal bone to the upper edge of the distal one. This should be measured at the maximum diameter and at right angles to the midline.

7. The *head circumference* (HC) can also be measured in this plane and is useful particularly at later gestations when there may be dolicocephaly (small BPD owing to elongation in the transverse plane) or brachycephaly (large BPD owing to widening in the transverse plane).

B. The transcerebellar (Fig. 3.4)

This plane is used to assess the posterior fossa structures which are the cerebellar hemispheres, connected by the vermis, and the cisterna magna. The fourth ventricle lies anterior to the vermis in the midline and is hardly seen.

1. In the transthalamic plane, fix on the cavum septum pellucidum and rotate the transducer into the posterior fossa until the *cerebellar hemispheres* come into view.

2. Check the shape of the cerebellum which appears like the double-headed *dumb-bell* used in weight training. A cerebellum which is banana shaped is associated with spina bifida.

3. Measure the *transcerebellar distance* (TCD) from the outer edge of one hemisphere to the outer edge of the other. This measurement in millimetres correlates with gestational age from 15 to 25 weeks when the cerebellum is easily visualised. Hypoplasia may be associated with spina bifida.

4. Look at the *cisterna magna* which is the subarachnoid space posterior to the cerebellum filled with CSF. It usually measures no greater than 10 mm but care must be taken with this measurement which can be falsely enlarged with too much angulation of the probe. It is usually very enlarged when associated with pathology as in the Dandy–Walker malformation when there is absence of the vermis and cerebellar hypoplasia.

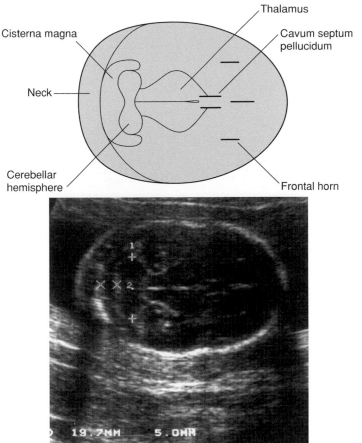

Cisterna magna

Neck

Cerebellar
hemisphere

Thalamus

Cavum septum
pellucidum

Frontal horn

Fig. 3.4 *The transcerebellar plane.*

C. The transventricular (Fig. 3.5)

This plane is used to assess the lateral cerebral ventricles to determine if there is enlargement (ventriculomegaly) or choroid plexus cysts.

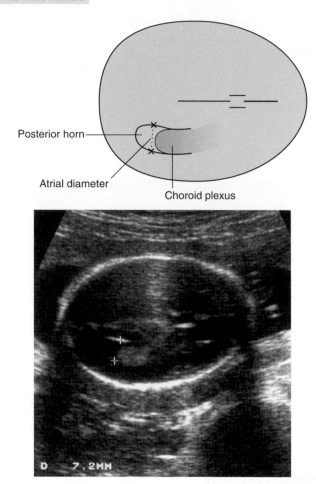

Fig. 3.5 *The transventricular plane.*

1. From the transthalamic view, move the transducer in the same transverse plane towards the vault of the skull until the *choroid plexus* is identified in the ventricle further from the probe. The proximal choroid plexus and ventricle are always less clear. You should find the choroid plexus arising from the medial wall of the ventricle and extending into the posterior horn. It normally occupies the width of the ventricle.

2. Identify the medial and lateral borders of the atrium running parallel to the midline. Make sure the view is transverse and measure the *atrial diameter* perpendicular to the axis of the ventricle. More than 10 mm is regarded as ventriculomegaly (Fig. 3.6). If there is gross enlargement of the ventricles, the choroid plexus will appear like the clapper of a bell in the distal ventricle because it is gravity dependent (Fig. 3.7). There are many causes of ventriculomegaly and they can be classified as outlined in Box 3.1 (see also Figs 3.8, 3.9).

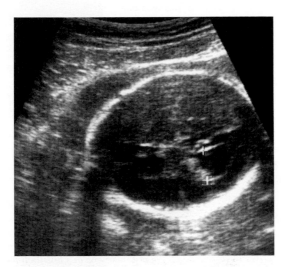

Fig. 3.6 Ventriculomegaly (atrial diameter = 13.7 mm).

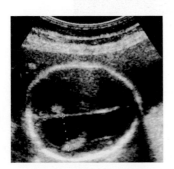

Fig. 3.7 The atrial diameter measured 17 mm in keeping with gross ventriculomegaly or hydrocephaly.

Fig. 3.8 *Hydrocephaly and no midline echo in keeping with alobar holoprosencephaly.*

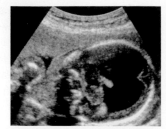

Fig. 3.9 *Obvious dilatation of the lateral ventricles and the third ventricle. This was due to aqueduct stenosis (see Fig. 3.1).*

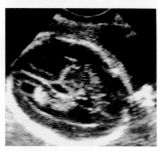

Case Scenario (Fig. 3.10A, B)

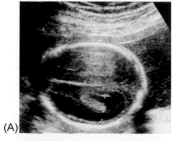

(A)

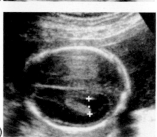

(B)

This patient was referred because of suspected ventriculomegaly, the atrial measurement being 14 mm **(A)**. However, the inferior caliper had been placed in the wrong position. **(B)** shows the correct placement of the inferior caliper, giving a measurement of 8 mm which is less than the upper limit of 10 mm. Be careful not to make this understandable mistake.

The orbits (Fig. 3.11)

From the transthalamic plane, rotate the transducer in the opposite direction to that which you selected to view the cerebellar hemispheres. You can now visualise the bony orbits and the hypoechoic lenses. At 20 weeks, the distance between the orbits (interorbital diameters) is similar to that of the orbit itself (ocular diameter). In certain instances you may wish to measure these, as well as the binocular distance from the outer aspect of one orbit to that of the other, and reference graphs can be used. Hypertelorism refers to the orbits being too far apart and hypotelorism is the opposite.

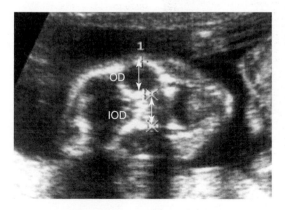

Fig. 3.11   *The orbits: ocular diameter (OD) = 11.2 mm; interorbital diameter (IOD) = 11.5 mm.*

The lips (Fig. 3.12)

From the transthalamic plane, rotate the transducer 90 degrees to obtain a coronal section and then move the transducer anteriorly to the face. Slight tilting will be required to view the lips. In this view, you may find cleft lip (Fig. 3.13).

You may wish to obtain a profile view of the face seen on sagittal section. This view is used in circumstances where a small jaw may be suspected (micrognathia). However, your departmental policy will dictate the time you have allocated for a detailed scan and routine visualisation of the facial profile and the ears is time-consuming and not usually feasible.

The neck

This is not normally seen as a separate entity unless there is a cystic or solid swelling and this is usually easily detected (Fig. 3.14).

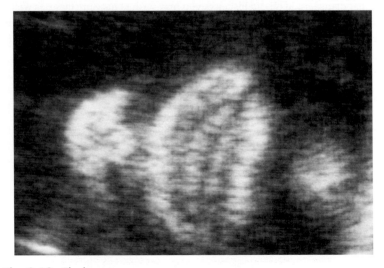

Fig. 3.12 *The lips.*

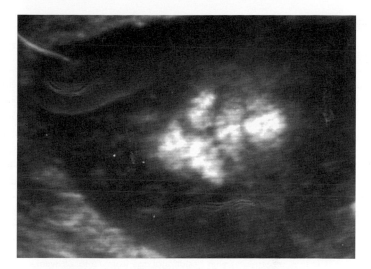

Fig. 3.13 Cleft lip.

Case Scenario (Fig. 3.14)

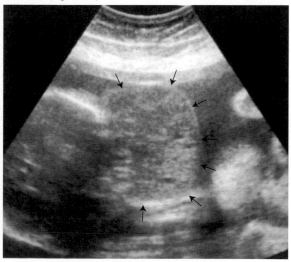

This solid neck tumour was detected at the time of a 20-week detailed scan. The mother subsequently developed polyhydramnios and went into preterm labour. The baby died soon after delivery secondary to tracheal hypoplasia and compression.

Checklist for head

Oval outline
Thalami
Short falx
Cavum septum pellucidum
Measure BPD, HC
Dumb-bell cerebellar hemispheres

Measure TCD
Assess cisterna magna
Choroid plexus
Atrial diameter
Orbits
Lips

Points to remember

1. The BPD has an accuracy within 5–10 days between 13 and 22 weeks. After this time, assessment of gestational age is much less accurate.
2. The TCD in mm correlates with gestational age from 15 to 25 weeks.
3. The cisterna magna normally measures no more than 10 mm.
4. An atrial diameter more than 10 mm is in keeping with ventriculomegaly.
5. At 20 weeks, the interorbital diameter is similar to the ocular diameter.

3.2

The spine

The most common lesion to affect the spine is spina bifida where there is failure of the dorsal portions of the spine to fuse. It is more common in the lumbosacral region. There are several variations and predicting severity is difficult because movement of the lower limbs does not equate to function. Classification into four categories is helpful (Fig. 3.15):

a. spina bifida occulta – the defect is covered by skin and may be identified by a tuft of hair. It is not detectable ultrasonically and there is usually no neurological involvement.

b. meningocele – there is a herniation of the meninges through the defect and there is a skin covering but there is no neural tissue.

c. myelomeningocele – there is a herniation of the meninges with involvement of neural tissue and the defect is usually covered by a thin membrane.

d. myelocele – this is the most extreme where there has been failure of the neural groove to close with consequent exposure of neural tissue.

With myelomeningoceles there is usually caudal displacement of the medulla and cerebellum resulting in obstruction of the foramen magnum and the development of hydrocephaly (the Arnold–Chiari malformation). These result in the head signs seen on ultrasound.

Examination of the fetal spine involves visualising the three primary ossification centres of the vertebrae and the skin covering the spine. The ossification centres are located in the body of each vertebra (central) and at the base of each transverse process (posterolateral) (Fig. 3.16). They are all visible by 20 weeks apart from those in the sacrum which may not appear until after 22 weeks. The spines of the vertebrae are not visible.

1. Always undertake your examination of the brain before proceeding to the spine because therein lie the clues to spina bifida – lemon sign (Fig. 3.17), banana sign (Fig. 3.18), ventriculomegaly (Figs 3.6, 3.17), small BPD and cerebellum, obliteration of the cisterna magna. It is helpful to know the serum alphafetoprotein (AFP) value at 16–20 weeks. If it is less than two multiples of

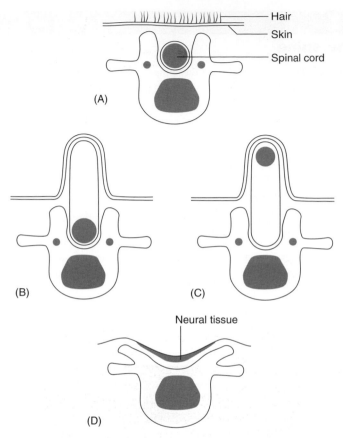

Labels in figure:
- Hair
- Skin
- Spinal cord
- (A)
- (B)
- (C)
- Neural tissue
- (D)

Fig. 3.15 *Types of spina bifida:* **(A)** *spina bifida occulta;* **(B)** *meningocele;* **(C)** *myelomeningocele;* **(D)** *myelocele.*

the median, there is less than a 1 in 1000 chance that the fetus could have an open neural tube defect.

2. Obtain a longitudinal view of the fetus and, concentrating on the spine, move your transducer to obtain a parasagittal view and confirm the *integrity of the skin* covering the length of the spine (Figs 3.19, 3.20). In this view you will also see the central and one of the posterolateral ossification centres.

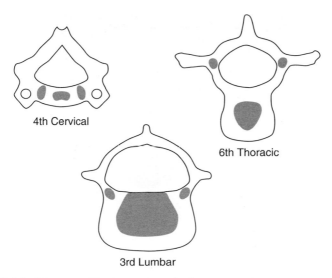

Fig. 3.16 Primary ossification centres of spine.

4th Cervical

6th Thoracic

3rd Lumbar

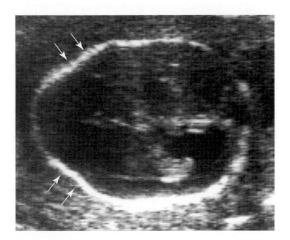

Fig. 3.17 Lemon sign and obvious dilated cerebral ventricle.

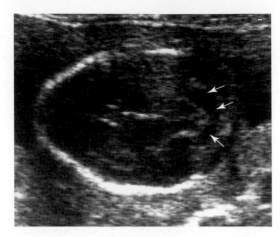

Fig. 3.18 *Banana sign.*

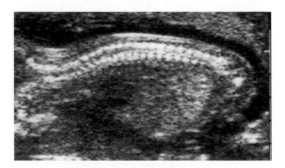

Fig. 3.19 *Integrity of skin (parasagittal plane).*

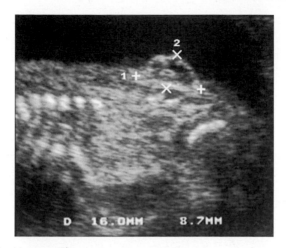

Fig. 3.20 *Meningocele.*

3. Now rotate your transducer to 90 degrees and, beginning at the cervical spine, view the vertebrae in this transverse plane along the length of the spine. Visualise the *ossification centres* which *normally appear closed around the spinal cord* (Fig. 3.21). If a defect is present you will find significant divergence of the lateral ossification centres (Fig. 3.22) and you may identify a protruding sac (meningocele).

4. Complete your examination and view the coronal plane to obtain the *railtrack appearance* of the ossification centres with the posterolateral centres being parallel to one another (Fig. 3.23). With spina bifida, which is more common in the lumbosacral region, there is splaying of the posterolateral ossification centres. Be careful not to over-diagnose because there is normally obvious widening in the upper cervical spine near the head and very slight widening in the lumbar region.

5. Always check the base of the spine where a sacrococcygeal teratoma may originate, usually as a large structure with irregular echo-bright areas (Fig. 3.24).

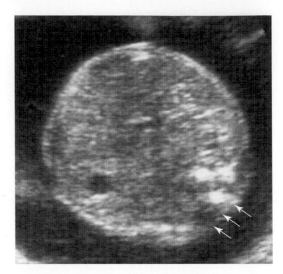

Fig. 3.21 *Ossification centres closed around spine.*

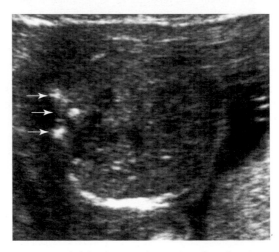

Fig. 3.22 *Open spina bifida showing divergence of ossification centres.*

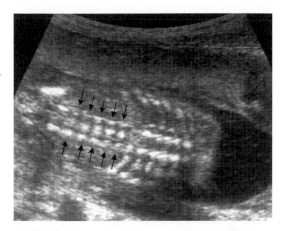

Fig. 3.23 *Coronal view of intact lumbar spine (railtrack appearance).*

Case Scenario (Fig. 3.24)

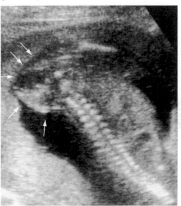

This woman attended for a detailed fetal scan at 20 weeks. The spine was seen to be intact but there was a solid 4 × 4 cm mass with cystic areas arising from the sacral area. The findings were in keeping with a sacrococcygeal teratoma. The patient went into preterm labour at 35 weeks and had a normal delivery. The tumour was successfully resected.

Checklist when looking at spine

Head shape, ventricles, posterior fossa, (AFP)
Railtrack appearance on coronal view
Skin intact on parasagittal view
Ossification centres closed around spine in transverse plane

Points to remember

1. There are three primary ossification centres visible.
2. Spina bifida is more common in the lumbosacral region.
3. There is normally obvious widening of the upper cervical spine and, to a lesser extent, the lumbar spine.

The chest

You need to check the four-chamber heart, its outflow tracts, the lung fields and the diaphragm. You require to understand the fetal circulation which will help you understand the anatomy of the heart. Follow the passage of blood from the placenta.

The fetal circulation (Fig. 3.25)

Blood enters the fetal heart from the inferior and superior vena cavae into the right atrium. Much of this blood is oxygenated, having come from the placenta through the umbilical vein via the ductus venosus in the liver to the inferior vena cava. The fetal lungs are not required for oxygenation of the blood, most of which passes from the right atrium into the left atrium via the patent foramen ovale and then to the left ventricle and out through the aorta. The blood which reaches the right ventricle from the right atrium passes out through the pulmonary artery and returns into the aorta via the ductus arteriosus. A small component returns through the pulmonary veins. At birth the ductus venosus, the foramen ovale and ductus arteriosus normally close as a consequence of the flow and pressure changes from the closure of the umbilical vein and arteries.

The heart and outflow tracts

To visualise the four chamber view and outflow tracts, there are five standard views which ensure a systematic examination. These mainly transverse views are obtained by moving from the inferior to superior regions of the fetal thorax (Fig. 3.26). It is the most difficult part of the detailed anomaly scan and will take you longer to master than anything else. The echocharity foundation (echo[UK], www.echocharity.org.uk) has produced pictorial charts of these views and it is useful to have one on the wall of your office or scanning room for easy recall. The charity offers training and education materials. It promotes the five transverse views and, with kind permission, has allowed us to reproduce the diagrams and images (Figs 3.26–3.31).

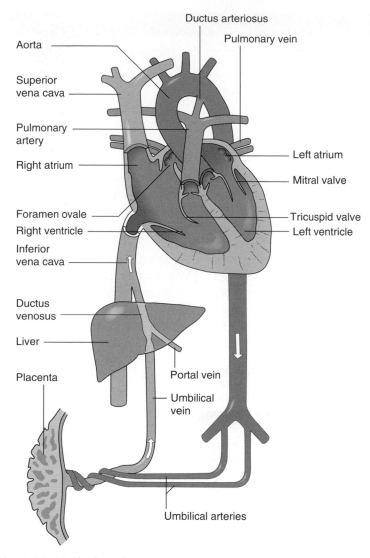

Fig. 3.25 *The fetal circulation.*

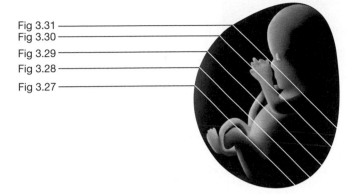

Fig 3.31
Fig 3.30
Fig 3.29
Fig 3.28
Fig 3.27

Fig. 3.26 *The five transverse views. (Reproduced with kind permission from www.echocharity.org.uk and Siemens Medical Solutions.)*

Orientation (Fig. 3.27)

1. Determine the lie of the fetus and obtain a transverse view across the abdomen to identify the stomach bubble which lies on the left (unless there is the rare occurrence of situs inversus).

Four chamber view (Fig. 3.28)

2. Maintaining the transverse plane, slide the transducer towards the fetal chest and visualise the heart pulsating and *four chamber heart* view. Slight angulation

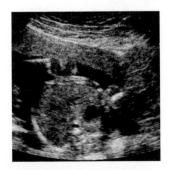
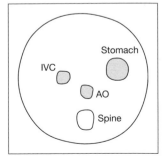

Fig. 3.27 *Abdominal situs, showing the position of the stomach, spine, abdominal aorta (AO) and inferior vena cava (IVC). (Reproduced with kind permission from www.echocharity.org.uk and Siemens Medical Solutions.)*

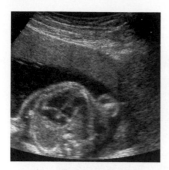
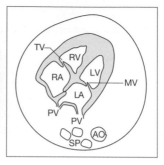

Fig. 3.28 *The four chambers, showing the connections of the atria and ventricles and the offsetting of the tricuspid valve (TV) and mitral valve (MV). AO, abdominal aorta; LA, left atrium; LV, left ventricle; PV, pulmonary vein; RA, right atrium; RV, right ventricle; SP, spine. (Reproduced with kind permission from www.echocharity.org.uk and Siemens Medical Solutions.)*

of the transducer towards the fetal head will help. Check that the apex of the heart and fetal stomach are on the same side and that the heart occupies about one-third of the heart area.

3. Identify the *left atrium*, which is the chamber nearest the fetal spine, and the *right ventricle*, which is nearest the anterior chest wall. Thus the right and left sides are identified with the long axis pointing to the left and the heart occupying about one-third of the thoracic cavity.

4. Check that the *atria* appear equal in size and, similarly, the *ventricles* and their muscle walls. At the apex of the right ventricle there is a bridge of muscle known as the moderator band which can make it appear slightly smaller. If in doubt, get it checked because this is the view to detect left or right heart hypoplasia.

5. Now look at the relationship of the *atrioventricular septum* and *valves* (the mitral is the left and the tricuspid the right). The appearance is that of a cross, slightly offset because the tricuspid is a little closer to the apex.

6. Check that the atrial and ventricular septa are intact. The interventricular septum is thinner near the valves (the membranous portion) and the interatrial septum is normally patent in its mid portion (the foramen ovale) where you

will see the flap valve opening in systole. Angling the transducer slightly towards the fetal head improves the image (the subcostal view).

Left outflow tract (Fig. 3.29)

7. Now with slight movement, move superiorly and angle the transducer towards the fetal right shoulder to look at the aorta emerging completely from the left ventricle. This is the *left ventricular outflow tract* passing across the aortic valve. It is visualised most easily when the ventricular septum is almost perpendicular to the ultrasound beam. The anterior wall of the aorta should appear continuous with the interventricular septum and the posterior wall with the anterior leaflet of the mitral valve.

Right outflow tract (Fig. 3.30)

8. Again with slight movement, continue rotating the transducer towards the right shoulder to obtain the long axis view of the pulmonary artery which heads posteriorly towards the fetal spine (*right ventricular outflow tract*). The pulmonary artery and aorta cross one another at their origins, with the pulmonary artery being more anterior and marginally larger. It courses posteriorly to the left and branches into the left and right pulmonary arteries and ductus arteriosus.

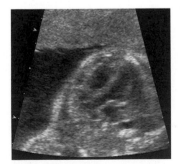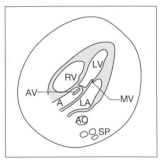

Fig. 3.29 *The left ventricular outflow tract, showing the aorta (A) as a continuum with the ventricular septum and travelling towards the right fetal shoulder. AV, region of aortic valve; other abbreviations as in Figure 3.28. (Reproduced with kind permission from www.echocharity.org.uk and Siemens Medical Solutions.)*

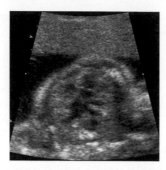
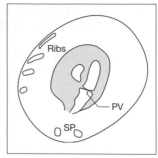

Fig. 3.30 *The right ventricular outflow tract, showing the pulmonary artery heading back towards the fetal spine (SP). PV, pulmonary valve. (Reproduced with kind permission from www.echocharity.org.uk and Siemens Medical Solutions.)*

Three vessel view (Fig. 3.31)

9. Now move superiorly to the fetal upper mediastinum. You are looking from right to left for the superior vena cava (in cross section), the transverse aortic arch and ductal arch (in longitudinal section), often remembered as dot, dash, dash. The aortic arch is directed posteriorly to the left and the ductal arch directly posterior. They meet at the descending aorta. The aortic and ductal arches should be equal in diameter.

If you have made it to here, have a rest.

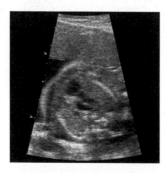
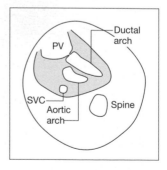

Fig. 3.31 *The three vessel view, showing the relationship of the pulmonary artery, ductal arch, aortic arch and superior vena cava (SVC). PV, pulmonary vein. (Reproduced with kind permission from www.echocharity.org.uk and Siemens Medical Solutions.)*

The lung fields

1. Return to the four chamber heart view to obtain a transverse view across the lung fields. Check *lung echogenicity* and exclude *fluid collections* and *cystic spaces*.

2. Lift and replace the transducer 90 degrees to obtain a sagittal view and look for the *diaphragm* which is seen as a thin line of low echo-density separating the abdominal visceral from the chest cavities (Fig. 3.32).

You should become familiar with the normal lung echogenicity. Any effusions gather peripherally in the pericardial and pleural cavities and are easily recognised (Fig. 3.33). Intrathoracic lesions may result in pulmonary hypoplasia and mediastinal shift (Fig. 3.34). If there is increased pressure on the venous return to the heart, pleural effusions and generalised hydrops may result. Increased external pressure on the oesophagus can lead to polyhydramnios.

Cystic spaces may signify a diaphragmatic hernia. Approximately 75% are left sided, 20% are right sided and 5% are bilateral. Left-sided hernias are easier to identify because the stomach bubble is displaced whereas, on the right side,

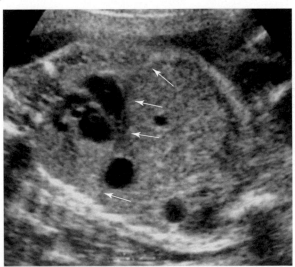

Fig. 3.32 *Echo-free thin line with stomach bubble (S) inferior in keeping with an intact diaphragm.*

Case Scenario (Fig. 3.33)

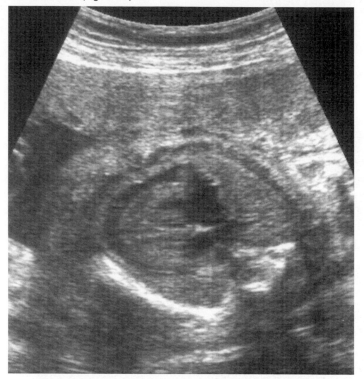

An echo-free area is seen demarcating the cardiac ventricles in keeping with a pericardial effusion. There was also mild ascites. Maternal serology revealed parvovirus infection. A repeat scan 1 week later revealed that the effusions had resolved and in utero blood transfusion for anaemia was not necessary.

the liver and small bowel have similar echogenicity to the lung. The observation of bowel peristalsis in the chest will confirm the diagnosis. The heart is frequently displaced. Sometimes defects in the diaphragm are not evident until after birth when the intrathoracic and abdominal pressures change.

More rarely, cystic spaces within the chest signify congenital cystic adenomatoid malformation (CCAM). CCAMs are due to bronchial atresia of varying degree. Ultrasonically it is best to describe the findings as macrocystic or microcystic. Macrocystic lesions may be single or multiple and are of varying sizes, all more than 5 mm. If there is associated hydrops and/or polyhydramnios, drainage of the larger cysts by needling or shunting may improve outcome. The main differential diagnosis is diaphragmatic hernia (Fig. 3.34). Microcystic CCAMs are less than 5 mm and appear as echo-bright solid lesions. If a lower lobe is affected, this may signify a bronchopulmonary sequestration where the lung tissue does not communicate with the bronchial tree (Fig. 3.35)

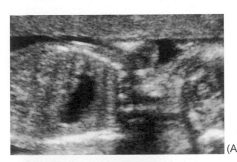

Fig. 3.34 **(A)** *Longitudinal and* **(B)** *transverse sections showing stomach in chest with mediastinal displacement. The findings were in keeping with a left-sided diaphragmatic hernia.*

(A)

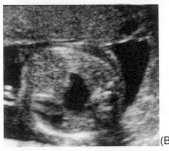

(B)

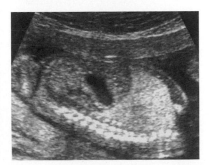

Fig. 3.35 *Hyperechoic lower lobe of lung. Postnatally this was found to be a pulmonary sequestration.*

Checklist for chest

1. Four chamber heart
2. Left atrium, right ventricle
3. Atria appear equal
4. Ventricles appear equal
5. Atrioventricular septum
6. Left ventricular outflow tract
7. Right ventricular outflow tract
8. Lung fields
9. No fluid or cysts
10. Diaphragm

Points to remember

In the normal four chamber heart view

1. The left atrium is nearest the fetal spine and the right ventricle nearest the anterior chest wall.
2. The ventricles appear equal in size, as do the atria.
3. The atrioventricular septum and valves appear as an offset cross.

In the normal view of the left ventricular outflow tract

1. The anterior wall of the aorta appears continuous with the interventricular septum.
2. The posterior wall appears continuous with the anterior leaflet of the mitral valve.

In the normal long axis view of the pulmonary artery

1. The pulmonary artery and aorta cross one another at their origins.
2. The pulmonary artery is anterior and marginally larger.

Artefacts

Moderator band.
Golf balls.
Membranous interventricular septum may appear as a defect.

Lung fields

1. Cystic spaces in a lung field signify a diaphragmatic hernia or a cystic adenomatous malformation.

The abdominal wall and contents

You now require to assess the integrity of the abdominal wall, the appearance of the kidneys, the renal pelves, the stomach, the bowel and bladder.

1. Obtain a transverse view of the *abdominal wall* to confirm its integrity and identify the *cord insertion* (Fig. 3.36). Such confirmation may be difficult when there is oligohydramnios causing distortion of the abdominal wall which may suggest exomphalos.

2. Establish that there is no central herniation in keeping with exomphalos and no lateral herniation to suggest gastroschisis (Fig. 3.37). With gastroschisis you will see a floating mass similar to a small bunch of grapes and initially it appears separate from the abdominal wall until closely inspected. The bowel is normally contained within the hernial sac in exomphalos (Figs 3.38, 3.39) whereas it floats freely in gastroschisis. They are associated with elevated

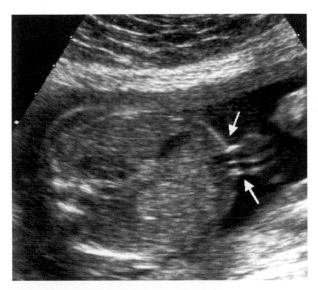

Fig. 3.36 *Abdominal wall with normal cord insertion.*

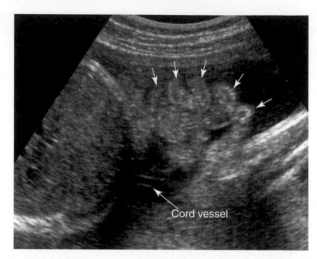

Fig. 3.37 *Loops of bowel seen in amniotic fluid lateral to the cord insertion. The bowel is not contained in a sac and the findings are in keeping with gastroschisis.*

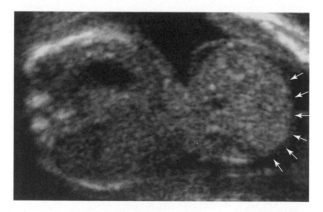

Fig. 3.38 *Anterior abdominal wall defect in keeping with exomphalos. The hernial sac does not contain liver or stomach.*

Case Scenario (Fig. 3.39)

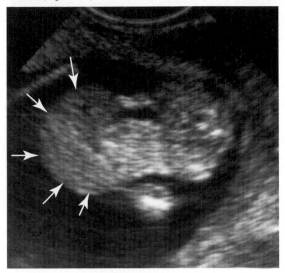

This transverse view of abdomen at 14 weeks revealed a large abdominal wall defect (19 × 22 mm) contained within an intact sac in keeping with exomphalos. A chorion biopsy was undertaken which revealed a 47XY+18 karyotype in keeping with Edward's syndrome. The patient opted not to continue with the pregnancy.

AFP. Exomphalos is associated with a chromosomal disorder in approximately one-third of cases (Fig. 3.39).

3. Now move to the upper abdomen maintaining the transverse view. Establish the presence of each kidney in its paravertebral position and visually assess the echogenicity (Fig. 3.40). Hyperechoic kidneys may be due to various pathologies. Unless there is a strong family history, the exact diagnosis is usually not made until after birth when further investigations can be undertaken. There are nomograms for the renal dimensions if you are concerned but any enlargement is usually gross and obvious (Figs 3.41, 3.42). Remember that the adrenal gland can mimic an absent kidney (Fig. 3.43). Familiarise yourself

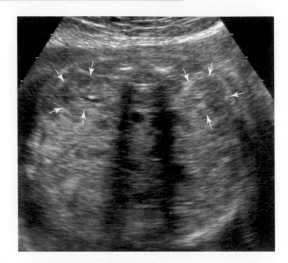

Fig. 3.40 *Normal kidneys and pelves.*

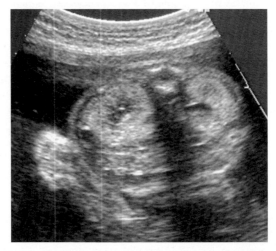

Fig. 3.41 *Enlarged echo-bright kidneys in keeping with multicystic renal dysplasia.*

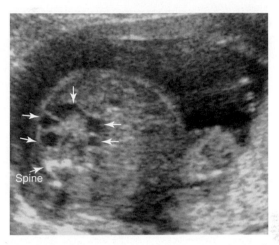

Spine

Fig. 3.42 *Unilateral multicystic kidney (an obstructive cystic dysplasia).*

with the four types of cystic renal disease encompassed in Potter's classification (Box 3.2). This gives an understanding of the pathogenesis.

4. Now look at the *renal pelves*. If you think they look dilated, measure the anteroposterior diameter. Mild dilatation (renal pyelectasis) of 5 mm or more (Fig. 3.44) is not uncommon and neonatal follow-up and investigation are necessary since one-third will have significant pathology. Gross dilatation of 10 mm or more is hydronephrosis and is always associated with pathology (Fig. 3.45). The potential sites of obstruction (functional or anatomical) should be considered. If you have found an abnormality of the collecting system, you should examine the bladder outline at this point to ascertain whether there is an obstruction proximal or distal to the bladder outlet (Fig. 3.46). The obstruction can be intermittent in nature and the exact pathology cannot usually be determined until after birth.

5. Having confirmed normality of the kidneys and their pelves, now move the transducer slightly caudally to check for the *stomach bubble* on the right side (Fig. 3.47). In this plane, you may see an echo-free rim which you may think is ascites. However, significant ascites is obvious and easily recognised (Fig. 3.48). Echogenic bowel as bright as bone may be found (see under 'soft

Case Scenario (Fig. 3.43)

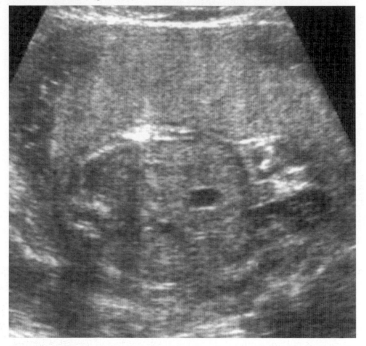

The above transverse view of abdomen at 22 weeks' gestation reveals absence of amniotic fluid. The differential diagnosis was considered. The possibilities were spontaneous rupture of the membranes, impending fetal demise or renal agenesis. A faint echo-dense outline can be seen on either side of the fetal spine which could be kidneys. However, the bladder was not visualised and a repeat scan 2 weeks later confirmed fetal growth but a bladder was still not visible. A diagnosis of renal agenesis was made and the parents opted not to continue with the pregnancy. Post-mortem confirmed the lethal condition of renal agenesis.

Box 3.2 Types of renal disease (Potter classification)

I Infantile polycystic
Autosomal recessive. Bilateral echo-bright grossly enlarged kidneys, oligohydramnios. Usually evident by 24 weeks but may be later.

II Multicystic renal dysplasia
Sporadic. Obstruction in early renal development. Unilateral or bilateral with multiple cysts of varying size.

III Adult polycystic
Autosomal dominant. Not normally detectable prenatally but may be suspected when there are enlarged echogenic kidneys, normal amniotic fluid and a parent with renal cystic change.

IV Obstructive cystic dysplasia
Sporadic. Later obstruction such as urethral valve or pelvi-ureteric obstruction. Unilateral or bilateral, small echogenic kidneys with peripheral cortical cysts.

Fig. 3.44 *Mild bilateral renal pelvic dilatation.*

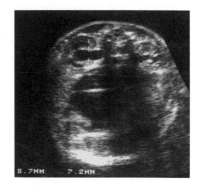

Fig. 3.45 *Unilateral hydronephrosis. The renal pelvic measurement was 12 mm.*

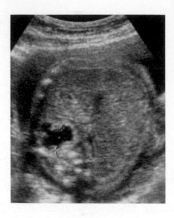

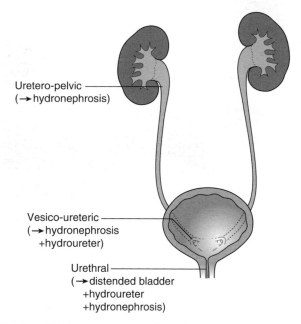

Uretero-pelvic
(→hydronephrosis)

Vesico-ureteric
(→hydronephrosis
+hydroureter)

Urethral
(→distended bladder
+hydroureter
+hydronephrosis)

Fig. 3.46 *Potential sites of renal tract obstruction.*

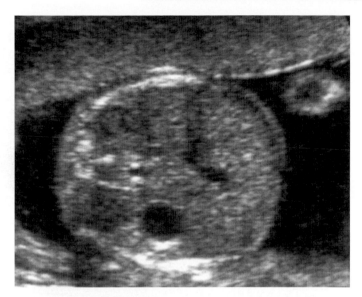

Fig. 3.47 *Normal stomach bubble.*

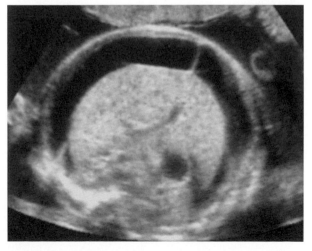

Fig. 3.48 *Significant echo-free rim in keeping with moderate ascites.*

markers'). Abnormal *dilatation of bowel* is not usually seen at the 20-week detailed scan and tends to be a later finding, often associated with polyhydramnios (Figs 3.49, 3.50, 3.51). Careful inspection is required when echo-free cystic areas are seen within the peritoneal cavity because they may arise from the renal tract or bowel, or be a simple mesenteric or ovarian cyst.

6. Now obtain a sagittal view to visualise the lower abdominal wall. Defects here are rare but are usually associated with bladder exstrophy and so confirmation of a *bladder* is important. Become familiar with normal bladder size. Emptying and filling can occur over 40 minutes. A hugely distended bladder is usually due to the posterior urethral valve syndrome in male fetuses (see also Ch. 2 on bladder outlet obstruction).

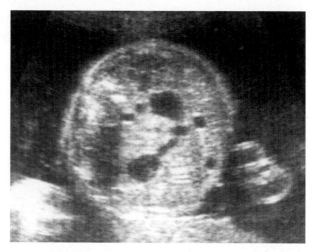

Fig. 3.49 *Transverse section of abdomen showing a double bubble in keeping with duodenal atresia. Approximately one-third are associated with trisomy 21 which was the karyotype found in this fetus.*

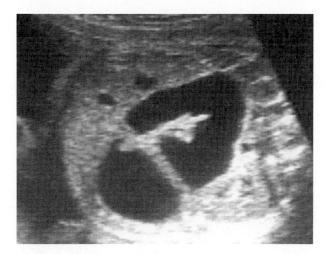

Fig. 3.50 Large dilated loops of bowel which at laparotomy after birth were found to be due to ileal atresia.

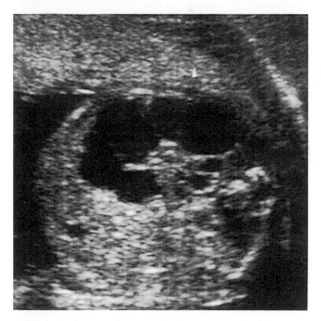

Fig. 3.51 Dilatation of fetal bowel at 24 weeks. Investigation of the parents revealed that they were carriers for cystic fibrosis and, following genetic studies on the amniotic fluid, the fetus was found to be affected.

Case Scenario (Fig. 3.52)

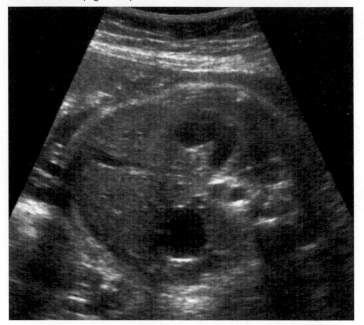

This transverse section revealed a double bubble which made the sonographer suspect duodenal atresia but in the parasagittal view visualisation of the kidneys revealed unilateral right-sided hydronephrosis. The echo-free areas seen in this section represent the fetal stomach and a dilated ureter.

Checklist for abdomen

Abdominal wall
Cord insertion and three vessels
Kidneys and pelves
Stomach bubble and bowel
Bladder

Points to remember

1. Exomphalos is a central defect, normally with an intact sac, and one-third are associated with chromosomal abnormality. Gastroschisis is neither.
2. Renal pelvic dilatation of 5 mm or more requires neonatal follow-up and investigation because one-third may be associated with pathology.
3. In renal agenesis, the adrenal glands may mimic the kidneys.
4. Dilatation of bowel is not usually seen at the 20-week detailed scan.
5. A double bubble may signify duodenal atresia and one-third are associated with trisomy 21.
6. Echogenic bowel may be associated with chromosomal abnormality, cystic fibrosis and infection.

The limbs

Measurement of the femur length (FL) is an essential part of the detailed scan. It supplements the BPD in assessment of gestational age. A measurement within the normal range excludes a lethal skeletal dysplasia (Box 3.3) and measurement of other limbs is not necessary. However, if below the normal range, then all limbs must be measured and assessed for mineralisation and evidence of fracture. In addition, the head and thoracic shape and size require evaluation. The differential diagnosis is a variant of normal, early intrauterine growth restriction (IUGR) (often caused by a chromosomal abnormality), or a skeletal dysplasia.

1. Obtain a transverse image of the fetal abdomen and move caudally until you reach the fetal pelvis and visualise the iliac crests. In this plane you will see an axial view of the femur.

2. Fix on the femur and rotate the transducer to obtain its full length. This is an important manoeuvre for you to master and develops your hand–eye coordination.

3. Try to obtain an image which is parallel to the top of the screen as this gives you the most accurate measurement of FL which is taken from the central endpoint of each metaphysis (Fig. 3.53).

Box 3.3 Lethal dysplasias

1. Thanatophoric dwarfism
Commonest. Obvious short bowed limbs, short narrow chest, clover leaf skull.

2. Osteogenesis imperfecta type 2
Obvious short long bones which are fractured.

3. Achondrogenesis
Obvious short limbs, short thorax, large head.

4. Camptomelic dysplasia
Mild shortening, bowing of femur and tibia.

Note. Achondroplasia is the second most common skeletal dysplasia but is non-lethal unless homozygous. The shortened limbs are not usually evident until the early third trimester.

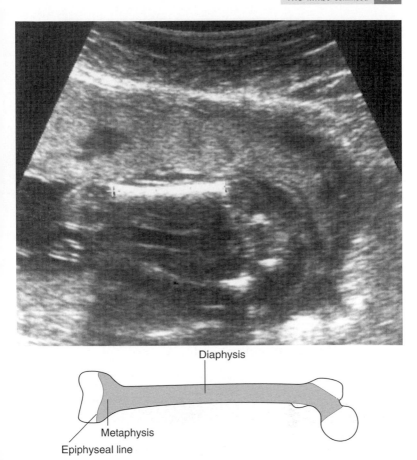

Diaphysis

Metaphysis

Epiphyseal line

Fig. 3.53 *Femur length measurement at 20 weeks. The femoral epiphyses are not seen by ultrasound until late in pregnancy and are not incorporated in the measurements.*

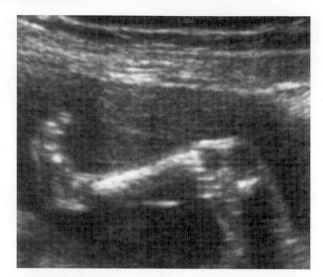

Fig. 3.54 Normal foot.

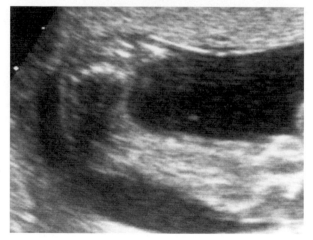

Fig. 3.55 Talipes.

4. Repeat the measurement twice or more to ascertain consistency. At 20 weeks, the femur measures 30 mm (range 25–35 mm).

5. Now move to the tibia and fibula to check their presence and relationship with the foot. Talipes is diagnosed when all the foot bones are seen in the same image as the tibia and fibula (Figs 3.54, 3.55).

6. Check the other leg for the bones and relationship to the foot.

7. Return to the transverse plane across the fetal trunk and move to the shoulder girdle. With similar manoeuvres, check for the presence of each humerus, radius, ulna and hand. These are not normally measured but tables are available if you are concerned. Identification of the fingers as a routine is difficult and time-consuming because the hands are clenched.

Checklist for limbs

Femur length
Presence of tibia, fibula
Presence and posture of feet
Presence of humerus, radius and hand

Points to remember

1. If the femur length is below the normal range, measure all limbs, evaluate head and chest.
2. Consider if normal variant, IUGR or skeletal dysplasia.

3.6

Soft markers

Soft markers are minor, usually transient ultrasonic features which have weak association with chromosomal abnormality. Most are not associated with structural abnormality. The initial reports came from referral centres suggesting strong links with chromosomal problems but these could not be extrapolated to the general population. The frequency of detection has been shown to increase with improved resolution of the ultrasound machine and with the expertise of the sonographers. Two or more markers are more strongly associated with an abnormal karyotype. Isolated choroid plexus cysts and cardiac echogenic focus should probably not be reported because they generate unnecessary anxiety. Your department will have a policy. The common markers are shown in Box 3.4.

Box 3.4 Common soft markers

Nuchal translucency (see p. 46)
Echogenic bowel (Fig. 3.56)
The echogenicity must be similar to or greater than surrounding bone. The finding may be a normal variant or associated with cystic fibrosis, cytomegalovirus infection, meconium ileus, trisomy 21, intrauterine growth restriction.
Choroid plexus cyst (CPC) (Figs 1.4, 3.57)
Folds of normal neuroepithelial tissue containing fluid and cellular debris seen as echo-free, well-circumscribed structures of varying size and number. Retrospective studies revealed up to 70% of trisomy 18 fetuses had CPCs. The reverse is not true. Isolated CPCs have a weak association with trisomy 18. Age seems to be the main risk factor. Available evidence has shown that at 32 years and over, the risk becomes greater than 1 in 250.
Renal pelvic dilatation (renal pyelectasis) (Fig. 3.58)
An anteroposterior renal pelvic diameter of 5 mm or more at less than 33 weeks and 7 mm or more thereafter. Definitions vary. Major benefit in identification of the fetus at risk of developing renal disease. The association with trisomy 21 is probably too weak to warrant intervention.
Cardiac echogenic focus (golf ball) (Fig. 3.59)
Located in the chordae tendineae not attached to the ventricular walls and seen to move with the atrioventricular valves. In the low risk population, not found to be associated with increased risk of trisomy 21.
Short femur and/or humerus
Fetuses with Down's syndrome are more likely to have shortened long bone measurements but an exact cut-off is difficult to define because of population and genetic differences.

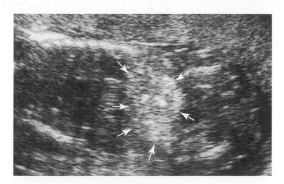

Fig. 3.56 Echogenic bowel.

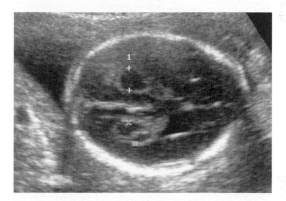

Fig. 3.57 Bilateral 7.5 and 7.2 mm choroid plexus cysts. As an isolated finding, these have a very weak association with trisomy 18 which is age related. Following this finding, the patient opted for amniocentesis for reassurance. The karyotype was normal.

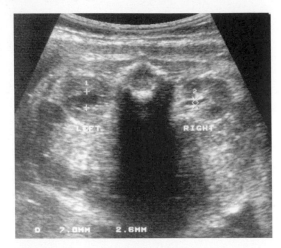

Fig. 3.58 *Mild unilateral renal pelvic dilatation.*

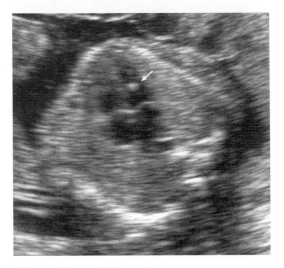

Fig. 3.59 *Echogenic focus in left ventricle*

The cervix, placenta and amniotic fluid

The cervix

The two main indications to visualise the cervix during pregnancy are to determine the relationship of the internal cervical os to the lower margin of the placenta (see p. 126) and to measure the cervical length in patients at risk of preterm labour.

When the cervical length is more than 30 mm, there is no risk of preterm labour. However, smaller measurements correlate poorly with the onset of labour. When the cervix is less than 20 mm (Fig. 4.1), 70% of patients will deliver preterm but 30% will not. In most pregnancies, the cervix naturally shortens in the third trimester so shortening is less important then. Dilatation and funnelling of the internal os may be seen and the worst scenario is protrusion of the membranes through a dilated cervix. The relationship between shortening, funnelling and dilatation is not entirely clear but it may be a progression. Clinically the ultrasonic measurement of cervical length has been found the most useful. Management options are not clear but in mid-pregnancy the obstetrician may consider the insertion of a cervical suture and the administration of antibiotics, based on your measurement.

Transvaginal ultrasound is the only technique which can be used reliably to measure the cervical length. Digital examination underestimates the length by at least 1 cm and transabdominal ultrasound overestimates when the bladder is full (Fig. 4.2). Any dilatation of the internal os will be reduced by pressure from the transducer and from bladder filling. If the bladder is empty, the cervix is visualised in only about half of cases with transabdominal ultrasound.

The technique of transvaginal scanning is described in Chapter 7. To assess the cervix in pregnancy:

1. Ask the patient to empty her bladder.

2. Slide the probe into the vagina only a few centimetres and rock the probe in the anteroposterior direction to visualise the cervix.

Fig. 4.1 *Transvaginal scan showing measurement of cervical length = 15 mm.*

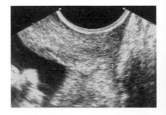

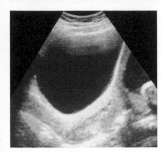

Fig. 4.2 *Transabdominal scan showing false elongation of the cervical length due to bladder filling. The measurement was 8.3 cm.*

3. Visualise the line of the internal cervical canal, remembering that it is not always a straight line.

4. Check that the anterior and posterior lips of the cervix appear equal.

5. Now slowly withdraw the probe a little and slide back to make sure there is no compression artefact.

6. Measure the cervical length from internal to external os. Record any funnelling which is generally accepted as membrane protrusion more than 5 mm down the canal.

7. Repeat the measurements three times and report the shortest.

Placental morphology

Embryology

A brief résumé of the embryological development of the placenta will help you understand the various ultrasonic appearances which are seen. The outer trophoblast of the embryo develops into the chorion when it implants into the maternal decidua and develops villous projections for gaseous exchange and the transfer of nutrients from the maternal circulation. This chorionic sac has a homogeneous appearance all round but, at about 9 weeks, differentiates into the chorion laeve (smooth) which becomes membranous, fusing with the amnion, and the chorion frondosum (frond-like) which becomes the true placenta (Fig. 4.3). The villi further invade the decidua which also proliferates with a vast network of endometrial veins and spiral arteries carrying maternal blood. With this invasion and proliferation, the placenta becomes septated by the decidua into segments called cotyledons and, within these, a vascular network develops on the fetal side (Fig. 4.4). Oxygenated blood from the placenta goes via the umbilical vein to the fetus and it returns via the two umbilical arteries for replenishment.

As tissue grows and develops within this vascular network, it is not surprising that occasional haemorrhage occurs. In addition, fibrin is deposited within

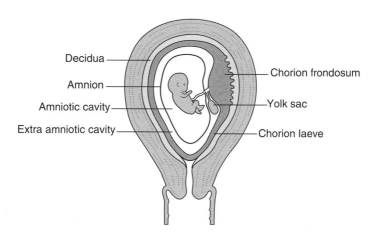

Fig. 4.3 Chorion laeve and frondosum.

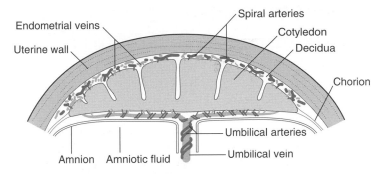

Fig. 4.4 *The placental circulation.*

the vascular channels, with resulting thrombosis and infarction to a varying degree, but when this is excessive, placental exchange will diminish to such an extent as to affect fetal growth and wellbeing.

Ultrasound appearances

When you scan the placenta you may be alarmed to see holes, bright spots and irregular lines. These appearances are extremely varied and, in isolation, are not closely linked with fetal compromise. The holes appear as focal hypoechoic areas and are simply venous lakes of blood (Fig. 4.5). The bright spots and irregular lines are evidence of calcification which is a result of normal degenerative changes seen in the third trimester. The lines eventually delineate the cotyledons (Fig. 4.6). Their prognostic significance is unknown but may be of concern before 34 weeks. Excessive calcification may be associated with a small fetus and pre-eclampsia but its significance in isolation is unknown.

You may think the placenta looks excessively thick or thin. A very small placenta may be associated with growth restriction. More than 3 cm thickness before 20 weeks and more than 5 cm before 40 weeks is considered abnormal. An excessively large placenta may be associated with infection, anaemia or triploidy and there are usually other markers of fetal compromise.

When you scan behind the placenta and at its edges, you may see large dilated vessels as great as 1 cm diameter. This is a normal finding and simply reflects the maternal vascular network of endometrial (or spiral) arteries and veins (Fig. 4.7).

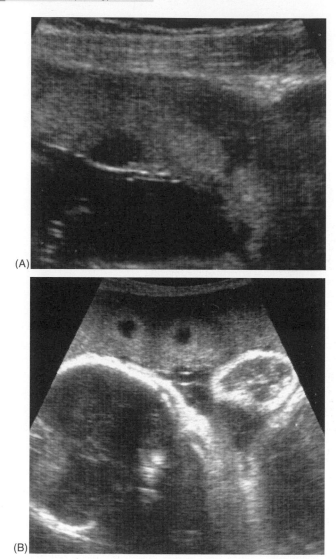

Fig. 4.5 (A,B) *Placental venous lakes.*

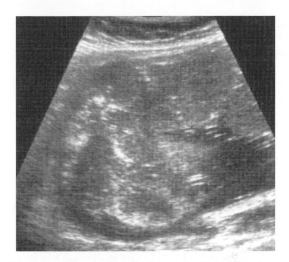

Fig. 4.6 *Placental calcification seen at 36 weeks. Not reported, since clinical significance at this gestation is unknown.*

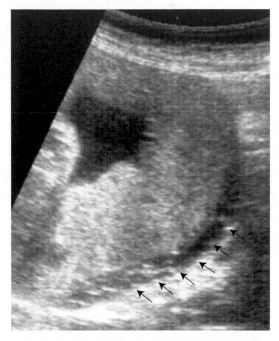

Fig. 4.7 *Maternal vascular network of endometrial arteries and veins.*

Antepartum haemorrhage

Antepartum haemorrhage, bleeding from the genital tract at or after 24 weeks, is a common problem in obstetrics. Vaginal bleeding before 24 weeks, the gestational age of viability, is classically referred to as a threatened miscarriage. You must have a working knowledge of the possible clinical causes (Box 4.1). If the blood loss has been excessive, it is likely that management will be dictated on the labour ward. The obstetrician will be using clinical judgement but the main differential diagnoses are placenta praevia or abruption (separation) of the placenta. Ultrasound is very helpful in the diagnosis of placenta praevia but less so for abruption. In the majority of patients, the cause will not be found and is often attributed to bleeding from endometrial vessels on the margin of the placenta. All such patients will be referred for ultrasonic assessment of the fetus and placenta. When the bleeding has settled, speculum examination will be undertaken to exclude any local causes.

Box 4.1 Clinical causes of antepartum haemorrhage

Placenta praevia (painless, soft uterus, high-presenting part)
Abruptio placentae (painful, tender uterus)
Vasa praevia (rare)
Local causes (e.g. cervical lesion)
Unknown or indeterminate (most common)

Placenta praevia – clinical and ultrasonic considerations

The classical clinical features of a patient presenting with placenta praevia are painless bleeding, a soft uterus with a high-presenting part or an oblique or transverse lie. The blood loss is mainly maternal. Historically, placenta praevia is divided into four grades and this classification predated ultrasound (Box 4.2). Grades I and II are regarded as minor degrees of placenta praevia and Grades III and IV are major (see Fig. 4.8). Ultrasound has given clarity to this classification and the grades are really now obsolete in clinical practice. If ultrasonically the placenta is seen to be covering the os and clearly below the presenting part, it is referred to as a major praevia. Vaginal ultrasound has added a further dimension, enabling the distance to be measured between the lower margin of the

Box 4.2 Historical classification of placenta praevia

Grade I   – the placenta encroaches on the lower segment but does not reach the internal os.

Grade II – the placenta reaches the internal os but does not cover it.

Grade III – the placenta covers the internal os eccentrically.

Grade IV – the placenta covers the internal os centrally.

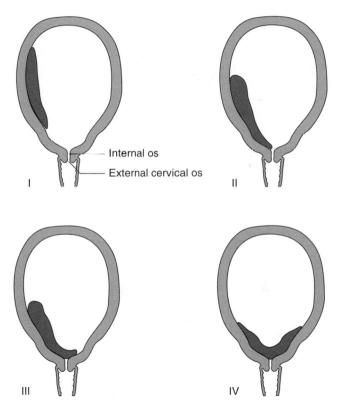

Fig. 4.8 *Grades of placenta praevia.*

placenta and the internal os. If the distance is less than 3 cm, then this should be regarded as in keeping with a major praevia. Distances of 3–5 cm are in keeping with a marginal praevia and such findings make clinical management difficult.

What the obstetrician wishes to know is whether or not the presenting part will be able to pass the edge of the placenta on its way through the birth canal without causing excessive bleeding. If the placenta appears to be obstructing safe passage, then it is likely that significant praevia is present and inevitable bleeding will occur.

Abruptio placentae – clinical and ultrasonic considerations

Abruption occurs when there is placental detachment and haematoma formation. The haemorrhage may be totally concealed with no vaginal bleeding occurring, or it may be revealed with no haematoma formation, or it may be mixed. The classical clinical features of a patient presenting with abruptio placentae are painful vaginal bleeding, a hard woody uterus and difficulty feeling the fetal parts. Both fetal blood and maternal blood are lost. In the extreme, the fetus will be dead or in distress in which case immediate delivery will be required. Such cases require intensive labour ward management and are not normally referred to your ultrasound department. Patients referred will usually have less striking clinical features. The obstetrician may be uncertain of the cause of the antepartum haemorrhage and normally wishes to exclude placenta praevia. Your ultrasonic assessment may reveal haematoma formation to suggest that an abruption has occurred.

Considering this background, proceed as follows:

1. Know the *clinical history*. Establish the gestation, the amount of bleeding and whether there was associated pain or not. The gestational age is important because the lower segment of the uterus is poorly formed before 34 weeks and a marginal praevia before this time can 'migrate' as the pregnancy advances. This is due to the progressive formation and elongation of the lower segment and the subsequent descent of the presenting part below the lower placental edge. However, a correctly diagnosed major praevia never changes. These occasionally do present clinically before 30 weeks but 10% of patients will have a low-lying placenta at 20 weeks (Fig. 4.9) and so it is better not to report a low placental location at the time of a 20-week detailed scan unless it is clearly centrally placed, occupying the lower part of the uterus. On the other hand, if the placenta is clearly fundal, then this is worth noting because it excludes praevia if the patient presents later with antepartum haemorrhage.

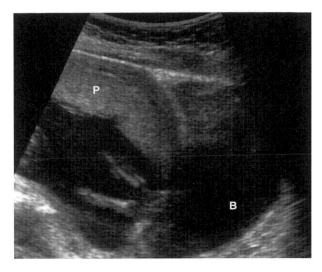

Fig. 4.9 *Low placenta reported at 20 weeks. A repeat scan at 34 weeks revealed the placenta to be in the upper segment confirming the prognostic inaccuracy of the earlier scan. B, bladder; P, placenta.*

2. Scan the contents of the uterus to determine the fetal *viability*, *lie* and *presentation*, and *amniotic fluid* volume. A high-presenting part may be associated with praevia. If the lie of the fetus is oblique or transverse, then interpretation of the placental location is difficult because the lower segment will be poorly formed.

3. Locate the placenta and move the transducer in the longitudinal plane to *delineate the lower edge*. You need to establish if it encroaches into the lower segment and, if so, its relationship to the internal cervical os and whether or not it lies below the presenting part. If you are suspicious, hold the transducer transversely and centrally over the lower segment and move it distally in this plane to identify the lower margin of the placenta. The lower segment is an anatomical entity which is difficult to define ultrasonically. A helpful landmark is the utero-vesical angle where the upper margin of the distended bladder meets the uterus (Fig. 4.10). This gives a rough guide to the upper margin of the

129

Case Scenario (Fig. 4.12)

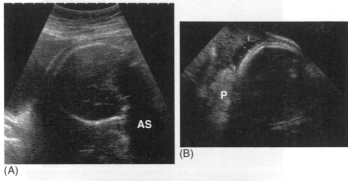

(A)

(B)

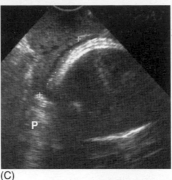

(C)

*The above scans were taken from a patient who was admitted with an antepartum haemorrhage at 34 weeks. The lower margin of the posterior placenta could not be clearly seen because of acoustic shadowing **(A)**. A transvaginal scan was therefore undertaken and revealed the placental edge to be 33 mm from the internal cervical os **(B)**. The patient was admitted and a repeat transvaginal scan was undertaken 2 weeks later which revealed that the placental edge was now 50 mm from the internal os with the progressive formation of the lower segment **(C)**. The patient was allowed home and went into spontaneous labour at 38 weeks and had a normal vaginal delivery.(AS, acoustic shadow; P, placenta.)*

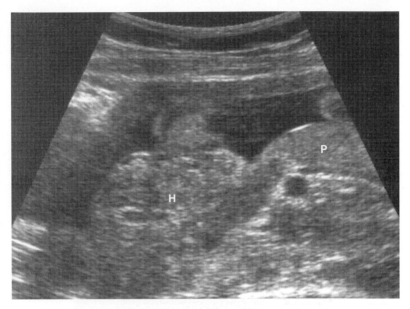

Fig. 4.13 *Echo-bright areas seen at the lower edge of the placenta in keeping with a marginal abruption. This may be confused with a low lying placenta. (H, haematoma; P, placenta.)*

4. Now look at the placenta to ascertain whether or not there is any *haematoma* formation to suggest that abruption has occurred. This is most commonly located at the edge of the placenta. Its ultrasonic appearance may be very similar to the placenta and sometimes difficult to differentiate (Fig. 4.13). The appearance will also change with time as the haematoma becomes organised and a mixed echogenic pattern may be seen. Less commonly, the haematoma may be totally retroplacental and may give the appearance of being within the placenta (Figs 4.14, 4.15). Rarely, a haematoma may appear subamniotic and preplacental (Fig. 4.16).

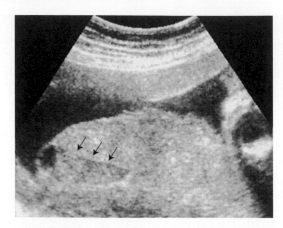

Fig. 4.14 *Area of mixed echogenicity seen within the placenta in keeping with a retroplacental haematoma. The patient was at 27 weeks' gestation and had vaginal bleeding and pain. The antenatal fetal heart rate pattern became abnormal and she required a caesarean section and an abruption was confirmed.*

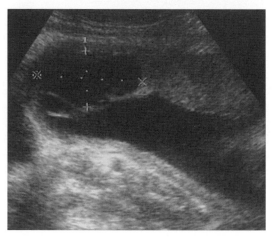

Fig. 4.15 *Echo-free area seen at placental edge. This was a resolving blood clot which had been seen as an echo-dense area 2 weeks previously.*

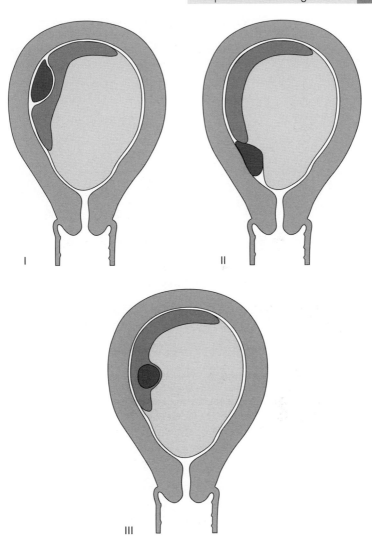

Fig. 4.16 Potential sites of placental haemorrhage: I, retroplacental; II, marginal; III, subamniotic, intraplacental.

Case Scenario (Fig. 4.17)

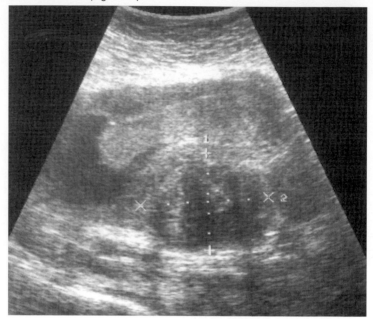

The sonogram on the above patient was taken at 20 weeks and revealed a 50 × 64 mm mixed echogenic mass which appeared to be behind the placenta. Initially, this was thought to be a retroplacental clot but on review of her case notes, it evolved that she had had a scan in a previous pregnancy which revealed a 50 × 50 mm posterior wall fibroid.

5. Check to make sure there is not a small lobe of separate placental tissue (*succenturiate lobe*) which may have vessels connecting it to the main placenta. When such vessels pass in the membranes in front of the fetal presenting part, they are termed vasa praevia and, if perforated, lethal fetal exsanguination can occur. This is rare. Colour flow imaging will aid identification.

Checklist for referrals with antepartum haemorrhage

Know clinical history
Determine lie, presentation, fetal heart pulsation, amniotic fluid
Delineate lower placental edge, consider transvaginal scan
Look for haematoma formation at edge, within or behind placenta

Points to remember

1. Retroplacental clot is an uncommon finding after the first trimester.
2. A lower placental edge within 3 cm of the internal os is in keeping with a major placenta praevia.
3. A lower placental edge 3–5 cm from the internal os is in keeping with a marginal placenta praevia.

4.4

Assessment of amniotic fluid

The regulation of amniotic fluid is not clearly understood. However, we know that in the first trimester, the main contribution is maternal and, thereafter, the fetus becomes progressively more responsible for its regulation. After 20 weeks, the main source of amniotic fluid is fetal urine and this is mainly cleared by fetal swallowing. Any disruption to these mechanisms will result in major changes in volume. The normal range is wide but approximate volumes are 300 ml at 18 weeks, rising to a maximum of 800 ml at 34 weeks, and falling to 600 ml at term.

There are three methods of assessment and your department will have a policy.

Subjective

> **Box 4.3 Subjective terms used to describe amniotic fluid volume**
>
> Virtually none (oligohydramnios)
> Reduced
> Average
> More than average
> Excess (polyhydramnios)

Sonographic experience of the average amniotic fluid volume is necessary before these descriptive findings can be used. Points to help you are:

1. The fetus occupies less than half the intrauterine volume up to 22 weeks.

2. The fetal abdominal wall normally is in contact with the anterior and posterior uterine walls in the third trimester and the fetal small parts are clearly seen, delineated by amniotic fluid.

3. Particulate matter may be seen floating in the amniotic fluid, especially near term. This is usually vernix or, sometimes, meconium.

4. *Oligohydramnios* may occur in the second and third trimesters. Although the fetal kidney starts functioning at 10 weeks, oligohydramnios is not seen until after 12 weeks. There are no pockets of fluid free of umbilical cord, there is crowding of fetal parts and hyperflexion (Fig. 4.18). Think of the possible causes (Box 4.4).

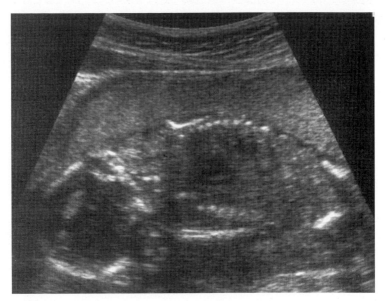

Fig. 4.18 *Oligohydramnios with crowding of fetal parts and hyperflexion. The cause of this was spontaneous rupture of the membranes at 20 weeks.*

Box 4.4 Causes of oligohydramnios

Idiopathic (usually less severe)
Ruptured membranes
Fetal abnormality causing reduced urine output
— renal agenesis
— polycystic kidneys
— urethral valve or agenesis
Placental insufficiency causing renal hypofunction
— intrauterine growth restriction
— postmaturity
— incidental

5. *Polyhydramnios* occurs usually in the third trimester. The views of the fetal anatomy, particularly the small parts, are very clear and the abdominal wall is surrounded by amniotic fluid. Again think of possible causes which your scan may detect (Box 4.5).

Box 4.5 Causes of polyhydramnios

Idiopathic
Macrosomia
Diabetes
Multiple pregnancy
Fetal abnormality causing impaired swallowing
— upper gastrointestinal obstruction
— neurological deficit (akinesia, myotonic dystrophy)
— other
Hydrops
Placental angioma

The terms 'reduced' and 'more than average' can lead to inappropriate clinical interventions. For this reason, objective methods have been devised to obtain a measurement which reflects volume. These are more reproducible and nomograms have been devised.

Objective

Measurements give a numerical value for the obstetrician and there is less inter-observer variation compared to subjective assessment. You must be careful not to apply too much pressure on the transducer because this will cause you to overestimate oligohydramnios and underestimate polyhydramnios.

A. Maximum vertical pool (MVP)

1. Scan the *whole uterine cavity* looking in particular between the fetal arms and legs, and around the neck for the deepest pool of amniotic fluid.

2. Locate the *largest pool* of amniotic fluid (minimum of 1 cm width) without limbs or umbilical cord and measure the maximum vertical distance (Fig. 4.19). When there is oligohydramnios, you may be fooled into believing there is a pool of amniotic fluid but this may contain only cord (Fig. 4.20). You can identify cord with colour Doppler.

3. If your measurement is reduced (less than 3 cm; Fig. 4.21), check and report on any *other pools* of liquor.

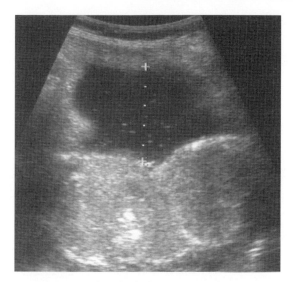

Fig. 4.19 *Maximum vertical pool. Flecks are seen in keeping with vernix.*

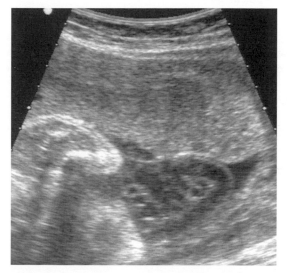

Fig. 4.20 *'Amniotic pool' containing cord – not measurable.*

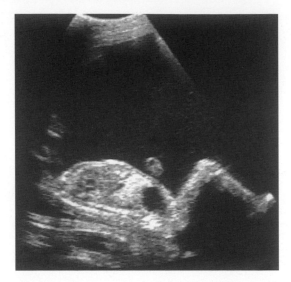

Fig. 4.21 *Obvious polyhydramnios in a case of twin-to-twin transfusion syndrome at 22 weeks. The deepest pool of amniotic fluid was 11 cm. Note the distended fetal bladder also.*

Box 4.6 Approximate values for maximum vertical pool measurements at 20–40 weeks

<2 cm	Oligohydramnios
2–3 cm	Reduced
3–8 cm	Normal
>8 cm	Polyhydramnios

B. Amniotic fluid index (AFI)

1. You require to locate the *largest pool* of amniotic fluid without limbs or cord in each quadrant of the uterus.

2. *Add* the measurements from each quadrant.

Box 4.7 Approximate values for amniotic fluid index measurements at 20–40 weeks

<5 cm	Oligohydramnios
5–10 cm	Reduced
10–20 cm	Normal
20–25 cm	More than average
>25 cm	Polyhydramnios

Checklist for amniotic fluid assessment

Scan whole uterine cavity
For MVP, locate largest pool and measure
For AFI, measure largest pool in each quadrant and summate

Points to remember

1. Amniotic fluid is formed by the mother until 12 weeks and by the fetus after 20 weeks. Between these times there is a progressive transition.
2. Oligohydramnios is defined as MVP less than 2 cm or AFI less than 5 cm.

Fetal growth and assessment

Indications

Requests for growth scans are frequent in the third trimester because clinical assessment may suggest that the fetus is too small or too large and most clinical complications (Box 5.1) which occur at this time may be associated with growth problems. A full fetal assessment is usually required including determination of placental site and amniotic fluid volume. The majority of patients have growth parameters within the normal range and such results reassure the clinician and patient. If the measurements suggest growth restriction, then cardiotocography (CTG) and Doppler studies will be required.

Box 5.1 Common clinical indications for growth scan

Small for dates
Large for dates
Pregnancy-induced hypertension
Antepartum haemorrhage
Maternal medical disorder (e.g. diabetes, lupus)
Preterm spontaneous rupture of membranes
Previous small baby

Normal growth

Environmental and genetic factors affect growth. The fetus increases in approximate weight from 500 g at 24 weeks to 1 kg at 28 weeks to 3.5 kg at 40 weeks. There is a rapid fetal weight gain from 27 to 37 weeks and then the growth velocity slows in the last few weeks (Fig. 5.1). It is during this time of rapid weight gain that serial scans for growth are appropriate and these are usually undertaken at intervals of 2–4 weeks depending on the clinical circumstances.

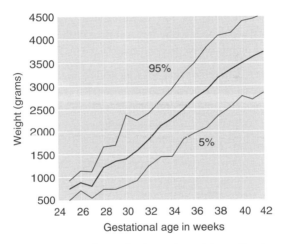

Fig. 5.1 Singleton birthweight centile charts derived from Aberdeen births, 1990–1997.

Case Scenario (Fig. 5.7)

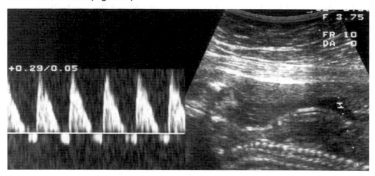

This Doppler flow pattern taken from the umbilical artery shows reversed end-diastolic flow. The patient had been admitted at 32 weeks with moderate pre-eclampsia. The AC measurement was just above the 5th centile and the amniotic fluid volume was normal. However, in view of the Doppler result, delivery was expedited. A live female infant weighing 1.47 kg was delivered by caesarean section and both mother and child made satisfactory progress thereafter.

In high risk pregnancies, umbilical artery Doppler assessment using absent or reversed end-diastolic flow has been proven to improve perinatal outcome. In low risk pregnancy, the use of routine umbilical Doppler assessment has been shown to be of no proven benefit.

The finding of absent or reversed end-diastolic flow is a rare finding in late pregnancy because the placenta is larger and a substantial degree of embolisation is required to prevent end-diastolic flow. Therefore, if absent or reversed end-diastolic flow is found after 34 weeks, delivery is warranted. When you find that end-diastolic flow is absent, make sure that this is not a false-positive result – it could be that the angle of insonation is too obtuse, at more than 60 degrees.

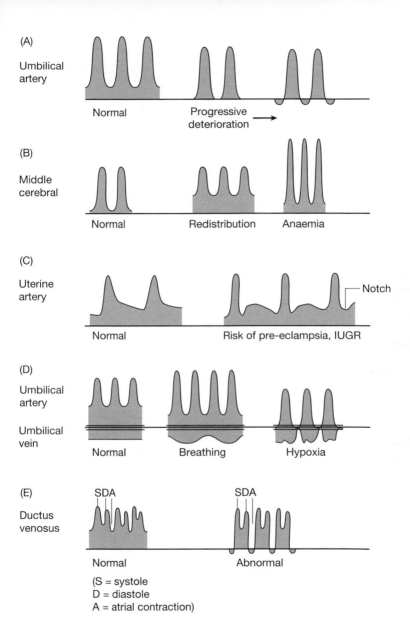

Fig. 5.8 *The various Doppler waveform patterns.*

(A)
Umbilical
artery

Normal

Progressive
deterioration ⟶

(B)
Middle
cerebral

Normal

Redistribution

Anaemia

(C)
Uterine
artery

Normal

Notch

Risk of pre-eclampsia, IUGR

(D)
Umbilical
artery

Umbilical
vein

Normal

Breathing

Hypoxia

(E)
Ductus
venosus

SDA

SDA

Normal

Abnormal

(S = systole
D = diastole
A = atrial contraction)

1. Identify a free-floating loop of cord and try to avoid sites adjacent to the placenta or fetal abdomen.

2. Using pulsed-wave (PW) Doppler, position the gate over the umbilical artery. The gate width does not affect end-diastolic flow but affects ease of detection of the signal.

3. Ensure that the Doppler angle is acute enough (<60 degrees is optimal), otherwise the trace will be small and inaccurate.

4. The thump (high-pass or wall) filter is used to remove the vessel wall movement during systole which can swamp the tracing. It must be set low, otherwise the end-diastolic flow will be cut off. Once set, it does not require readjustment.

Middle cerebral artery Doppler

There are two indications to measure middle cerebral blood flow.

A. To assess circulatory redistribution in severe IUGR

In the normally oxygenated fetus, there is low, absent and occasionally reversed end-diastolic flow from 20 to 28 weeks. It remains low from 28 to 34 weeks but increases thereafter. When fetal hypoxia occurs, there is an increase in the cerebral blood flow due to circulatory redistribution. This is seen as a reduction in the resistance indices with extensive end-diastolic flow being apparent (Fig. 5.8B). In severe hypoxia, an increase in resistance may be seen, 24–48 hours before circulatory collapse. This is thought to be due to cerebral oedema.

B. To assess fetal anaemia

Fetal anaemia may occur due to erythrovirus (previously known as parvovirus) or maternal isoimmunisation due to Rhesus, Kell or other antibodies. When this becomes significant, fetal cardiac output and blood flow velocity increase before hydrops develops. The measurement of the peak systolic blood flow in the middle cerebral artery has been shown to correlate well with the degree of fetal anaemia. This gives guidance as to when fetal blood sampling and likely transfusion are required. The measurement of bilirubin optical density of the amniotic fluid is no longer necessary to assess whether transfusion or delivery is required. This is a valuable technique to master.

162

1. From the transthalamic view, look for the echo-dense line of the wing of the sphenoid bone coursing anterolaterally.

2. Apply colour flow Doppler to visualise the vessels in the circle of Willis and the middle cerebral artery which courses along the sphenoidal wing (Fig. 5.9).

3. Apply pulsed Doppler perpendicular to the vessel close to the circle of Willis to obtain the waveform pattern.

4. Read off the maximum systolic velocity in cm/sec and plot on the chart (Fig. 5.10).

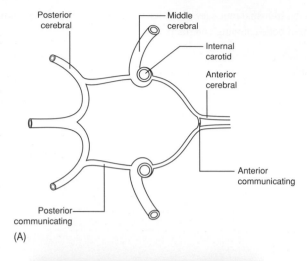

(A)

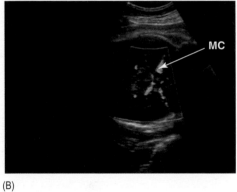

MC

(B)

Fig. 5.9 The circle of Willis.

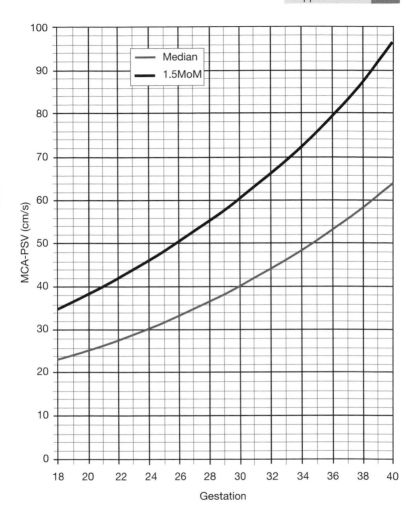

Fig. 5.10 *Chart of peak systolic velocity for middle cerebral artery.*
(Reproduced from Mari et al. N Engl J Med 2000; 341:9–14. Copyright © 2000 Massachusetts Medical Society. All rights reserved.)

Uterine artery Doppler

This is normally undertaken at 24 weeks' gestation. It has a role to play in the patient at high risk of pre-eclampsia. However, its diagnostic accuracy is only moderate in the prediction of pre-eclampsia and minimal for IUGR and perinatal death. There is no justification for its use in low risk patients.

The uterine arteries originate from the internal iliac vessels and approach the uterus at the level of the internal os. They ascend lateral to the uterine body and give off branches which penetrate the myometrium. These branches then divide into the so-called arcuate arteries which form a mesh throughout the outer myometrium. From these, radial arteries are directed to the endometrium and are visualised within the inner two-thirds of the myometrium. These pass through the myometrium and become the spiral arteries whose vessel walls become invaded by trophoblast during pregnancy. Due to this process, the spiral arteries become wide non-contractile channels and a compliant, low resistance intervillous circulation develops. This process is impaired in pre-eclampsia.

These physiological changes are reflected in the Doppler measurements taken from the uterine arteries. In the first half of pregnancy a 'notch' is characteristically seen between the systolic and diastolic flows due to high vascular resistance. The resistance decreases with advancing gestation and the notch should not normally be seen at 24 weeks (Fig. 5.8C).

A standard technique should be used to identify the uterine arteries and the use of colour flow Doppler improves reproducibility.

1. Using transabdominal ultrasound, place your transducer lateral to the uterus in the longitudinal plane to visualise the vessels in the pelvic side wall. Locate the external iliac artery and look for the uterine artery where it appears to cross over. You may find that it branches at or before the cross-over.

2. Using transvaginal ultrasound, place the probe in the anterior fornix and identify the cervix. Move the probe to the lateral fornix and identify the uterine artery at the level of the internal os.

3. Apply pulsed-wave Doppler and when a consistent waveform pattern is obtained, freeze the image and take the measurements.

4. The resistance is lower in the uterine artery on the placental side so you should repeat the resistance index measurements on the opposite side and take the average of the two.

When there is a high pulsatility index (average of left and right, >95th centile at 1.65) and/or bilateral uterine artery notches, there is an increased risk of pre-eclampsia and IUGR. It identifies around 40% of patients who will develop pre-eclampsia and 20% who will develop IUGR. Following a positive test, the likelihood of developing pre-eclampsia is sixfold. Closer monitoring of the pregnancy will then be required but there are no proven preventative measures which can be taken.

Fetal venous Doppler

This may be required to assess the fetus in the presence of severe early onset IUGR in the late second trimester and early third trimester. Oxygenated blood passes from the placenta to the fetus via the umbilical vein, the ductus venosus and the upper part of the inferior vena cava to the right atrium (Fig. 3.25). The lumen of the ductus venosus is much narrower than the umbilical vein and inferior vena cava, resulting in accelerated blood flow in this vessel. Certain changes have been associated with severe fetal compromise. You need to have colour flow and pulsed-wave Doppler on your ultrasound equipment to facilitate their interrogation.

The umbilical vein in the second half of pregnancy normally has continuous low flow velocity throughout the cardiac cycle and is non-pulsatile (Fig. 5.8D). Pulsations are seen in early pregnancy or when there is cord compression or fetal compromise. Low amplitude pulsations are associated with fetal breathing and assessment should not be undertaken during this phase. Pulsations reflect cardiac function rather than placental resistance. With cord compression, the pulsations occur during systole. Pulsations occurring at the end of diastole are ominous and indicative of severe fetal compromise.

The ductus venosus has accelerated blood flow and is closer to the heart, reflecting atrial function. It has a pulsatile waveform and three phases are seen (Fig. 5.8E). In the compromised fetus, the nadir due to back pressure from the atrial contraction increases, resulting in absent or reversed flow.

The inferior vena cava shows the same triphasic pattern as seen in the ductus venosus and reverse flow is frequently seen during atrial contractions so its value is of little use.

1. Identify the umbilical cord and the vein. If you wish to obtain umbilical venous flow, position the gate over the vessel, check that the angle of insonation is acute and obtain the flow pattern.

2. Follow the length of the umbilical vein through the fetal abdominal wall into the liver.

3. Using colour flow Doppler, identify the increased velocities at the end of the umbilical vein where the narrower ductus venosus originates.

4. Position the gate over the origin of the ductus venosus and adjust the beam angle to less than 30 degrees to ensure an adequate signal. It is helpful to listen for the hissing sound of the ductus venosus which distinguishes it from the nearby inferior vena cava and hepatic vein.

Checklist for umbilical artery Doppler

Free-floating loop of cord
Position gate over umbilical artery
Obtain an acute Doppler angle (less than 60 degrees)

Points to remember

1. The umbilical artery is the vessel which best predicts fetal condition.
2. The observation of absent or reversed end-diastolic blood flow in the umbilical artery is clinically more useful than the various indices.
3. Absent or reversed flow in the ductus venosus indicates fetal compromise.
4. Umbilical venous pulsations seen at the end of diastole indicate severe fetal compromise.
5. When there are bilateral uterine artery notches, there is an increased risk of pre-eclampsia and intrauterine growth restriction.

Biophysical profile

The biophysical profile is an assessment of fetal wellbeing. It is affected by factors which suppress the fetal central nervous system such as hypoxia, infection and maternal medication. It conveys a score (out of 10) for the obstetrician to gauge in the clinical context. A score of 2 is given for each component if the criteria are met and zero if not. The components are as follows:

1. *Fetal breathing.* Look for the rhythmic movement of the chest and abdominal wall which reflects that of the diaphragm and is easily recognised. You will see this as a prolonged episode lasting 30 seconds and it should occur at least once every 30 minutes.

2. *Fetal movement.* Look for significant body or limb movement and you should see at least three in 30 minutes. These of course can be assessed by CTG also.

3. *Fetal tone.* With this you need to assess flexion and extension movements of the body, limbs or hand. Look for arching of the spine, kicking or opening and closing of the hands and you should see at least one in 30 minutes.

4. *Amniotic fluid volume.* You should find at least one cord-free pool of amniotic fluid measuring 2 cm in two perpendicular planes.

5. *Antenatal cardiotocography* (CTG or non-stress test). A normal reactive tracing is one in which the fetal heart rate reacts with two or more accelerations to movements or contractions within a 20-minute period.

Modifications have been used relating to the amniotic fluid volume, and placental grading (see Ch. 4) has been incorporated by some.

The fetus has a sleep–wake cycle of 20–40 minutes and this is why the observation period can take up to 30 minutes. In the sick fetus affected by hypoxia or infection, the first markers to go are breathing and fetal heart rate reactivity and the last are movement and tone. Scores of 10 or 8 are reassuring, 6 or 4 are equivocal, and 2 or 0 are ominous. The aim is to identify when the fetus may require delivery before becoming seriously compromised.

The biophysical profile was introduced without randomised controlled trial evaluation to assess its benefit. Its main disadvantage is that it is time-consuming, taking up to 30 minutes to complete the scan and, in reality, it provides little additional information compared to a CTG and amniotic fluid volume. Therefore, in many centres it has now been superseded by CTG, amniotic fluid volume, growth and Doppler assessment. Your department will have its own policy.

Case Scenario (Fig. 5.11)

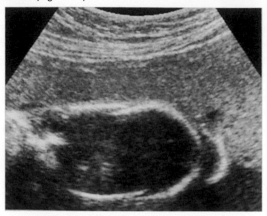

This patient was admitted at 26 weeks with reduced fetal movements for 48 hours and a scan confirmed an intrauterine death. This was totally unexplained. The image shows overlapping of the fetal skull bones (Spalding's sign) which is seen when death has occurred at least 24 hours previously.

Checklist for biophysical profile

Breathing movement
Gross body movement
Tone
Amniotic fluid
Reactivity of fetal heart rate

Points to remember

1. The biophysical profile is affected by factors which suppress the central nervous system.
2. A CTG and amniotic fluid volume assessment probably provide equivalent information.

Multiple pregnancy

Ultrasound is invaluable in the assessment of fetal growth in twin and higher order pregnancies. As in singletons, AC is the most useful parameter and this requires to be done serially to assess incremental growth. Twin growth charts have been derived and these are the same as for singletons up to 28 weeks after which time a slight tailing off occurs (Fig. 5.12). On average, you should find a 10 mm increase each week from 28 to 38 weeks. There are some tips on technique which you may find helpful:

1. The diagnosis of a twin pregnancy will usually be known from earlier scans. First, you require to determine the lie of each fetus and which one is leading. Start with your transducer held transversely in the lower segment area of the uterus to establish the presentation of the leading twin (twin 1). Now rotate your transducer to find the spine of this fetus and confirm a fetal heart pulsation. You will normally find that each twin is lying mainly to the right or left of the maternal abdomen. To find the second twin (twin 2), move back to the lower segment to establish the presenting part for the second twin. Find the spine and head of twin 2 and again confirm a fetal heart pulsation. You should by now have a mental map of the lie of each twin and be able to relocate the head and spine of each twin with ease.

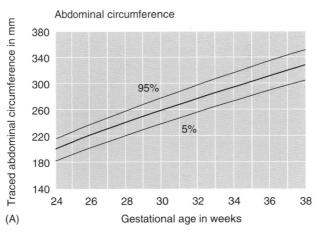

Fig. 5.12 *Twin growth charts derived from Aberdeen births.*

Continued

Biparietal diameter

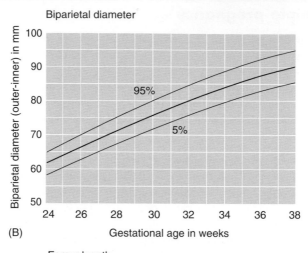

(B) Gestational age in weeks

Femur length

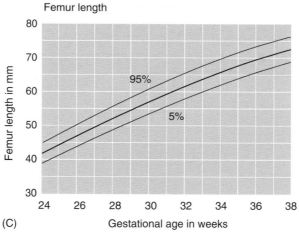

(C) Gestational age in weeks

Fig. 5.12 *Cont'd*

2. Now move back to twin 1 and undertake your growth measurements on this fetus and print them off. Now do the same for twin 2, keeping this set of measurements separately. By doing this in a set manner, you will avoid confusing which set of measurements come from which twin.

3. Report and plot your measurements and draw a map of the lie and relationship of each twin (Fig. 5.13). This will help orientation for the next growth scan.

You may find evidence of growth discordancy when there is an AC difference of more than 20 mm between each twin. Discordancy at birth is defined as the birthweight difference between the co-twins expressed as a proportion (or percentage) of the larger twin's birthweight. Differences in birthweight of 25% or more are associated with an increased perinatal morbidity and mortality in the smaller twin.

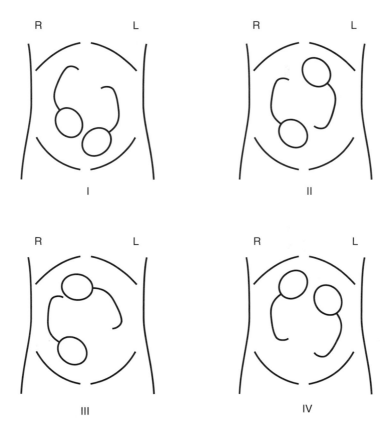

Fig. 5.13 *Mapping the lie and relationship of each twin.*

Once the diagnosis of discordancy has been made, then intensive fetal monitoring is required. In dichorionic pregnancies, this occurs as a result of growth restriction in one twin and in monochorionic pregnancies may be due to the twin–twin transfusion syndrome when the oligo/polyhydramnios sequence may develop.

The frequency of growth assessment will depend on the resources of your department but monochorionic twins require closer surveillance and we suggest 2-weekly scans from 20 weeks whereas in dichorionic twins, serial scans at 24, 28, 32, 35 and 37 weeks will suffice provided there are no ominous features.

Case Scenario (Fig. 5.14)

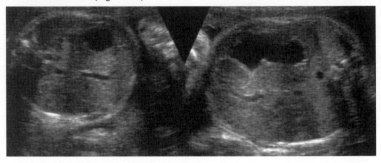

These images of the AC were taken from a set of dichorionic twins at 34 weeks' gestation showing marked discordancy, the AC of twin 1 measuring 231 mm and that of twin 2 measuring 287 mm. They had been monitored closely since 30 weeks when growth problems had first been detected. There had been no abnormal fetal heart rate patterns or Dopplers and the amniotic fluid volumes were normal in both. It is difficult to know when best to deliver and the balance of preterm delivery has to be weighed against the risk of intrauterine death. They were delivered at 35 weeks by caesarean section. Twin 1 was male and weighed 1.7 kg; twin 2 was female and weighed 2.5 kg. They were both admitted to the special care baby unit and made very good progress. The growth discordancy was 32% (2.5 − 1.7 ÷ 2.5 × 100).

Checklist for twin growth scan

Determine lie and relationship of each twin. Confirm viability
Undertake and record your measurements separately for each twin
Plot your measurements and sketch a map of the twins

Points to remember

1. AC is the most useful parameter to assess growth.
2. There is an average increase in AC of 10 mm per week.
3. Growth discordancy is present when there is a difference of more than 20 mm in AC between each twin.

Invasive procedures

Technique

It is standard practice to undertake all invasive procedures under ultrasonic guidance. This means that the needle tip is continuously visualised on its path to its intended destination. By this approach, you can ensure the safe passage of the needle and avoid unnecessary perforation of maternal or fetal structures. There is now no place in modern clinical practice for blind aspiration with its increased failure rate owing to inability to know the true location of the needle tip. There are two approaches to ultrasonic guidance:

1. *Biopsy needle guide*. You can attach a needle guide to your transducer and a guidance track (single or double lines) appears on the screen. There are markers at fixed intervals to give you measurements of depth which help you assess how far to insert your needle (Fig. 6.1). You may find this technique helpful when you begin to do amniocentesis. However, with the needle being

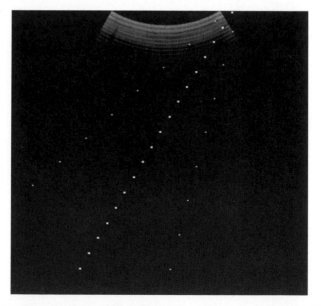

Fig. 6.1 *Biopsy guideline with depth gauge markers at 1 cm intervals. The needle follows the track of the central line.*

fixed, there is less scope for fine adjustment which is required for smaller targets. Some operators use the technique to guide them to the target area and then free the needle from the applicator to allow flexibility.

2. *Free hand technique.* This means that there is flexibility to move the needle freely and it is not restricted by the needle guide. This is a bimanual technique and coordination between both hands is essential so that the needle must be parallel and in line with the transducer to visualise its length and tip. Your right brain requires to know what your left brain is doing – the ultimate in coordination.

Look at your field and target on the screen and imagine the approach of your needle. The difficulty is knowing the exact angle to insert your needle and you can do this by first visualising and adjusting the local anaesthetic needle direction. The key is to adjust your needle path and align it to your target view because the latter is fixed. Place the needle 1–2 cm from the transducer and follow its passage on the screen. A curvilinear transducer with its splayed beam is best. Visualisation of the needle is optimum when it is at right angles to the beam. You may wish to move your transducer away from your insertion point to achieve this (Fig. 6.2).

As with all practical procedures, there is a learning curve and initially it is best to practise on fluid-filled plastic models. You should have an experienced

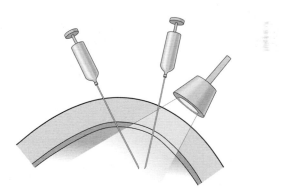

Fig. 6.2 *Visualisation of needle using the free hand technique. Insertion of the needle at 60 degrees close to the transducer or more distally at right angles to ultrasound beam.*

operator assisting you when you undertake your first 5–10 amniocenteses until your supervisor is satisfied with your technique and you feel confident. There should always be someone to assist if you are having difficulty. After you have undertaken 30 with success, you are competent and you should undertake about 30 per annum to maintain your skill. There is a progression of skill required for the subsequent procedures described below and this is related to the target size and mobility.

Amniocentesis

There are several reasons for undertaking amniocentesis (Box 6.1), the most common being to determine fetal karyotype and specifically to exclude trisomy 21 in older women. Some single gene disorders are best diagnosed from amniotic fluid but most are now undertaken using chorion. In establishing the severity of Rhesus isoimmunisation in the third trimester, the measurement of the optical density of bilirubin in the amniotic fluid has been replaced by middle cerebral artery Doppler assessment (p.162). In patients with painful polyhydramnios, serial amnioreduction can alleviate the discomfort and may prolong pregnancy. The measurement of amniotic fluid concentrations of alphafetoprotein and the detection of acetylcholinesterase to improve the sensitivity in making the diagnosis of neural tube and abdominal wall defects are now rarely required because of the improved resolution of ultrasound equipment. Similarly, accuracy of pregnancy dating from early ultrasound, advances in neonatal intensive care and the widespread use of corticosteroids have meant that the assessment of lung maturity from the lecithin/sphingomyelin ratio is no longer used.

1. Inform the patient about the procedure, the risk of miscarriage (0.5–1%), the reporting time for your service and the risk of failed culture (1%). The procedure should always be undertaken with ultrasound guidance to visualise needle entry into the amniotic cavity.

2. Perform an ultrasound scan to confirm gestational age and viability and to check the fetal anatomy. Elective amniocentesis for determination of karyotype is normally undertaken at 16 weeks. Before 14 weeks, the fetal loss rate is higher. This is due to the increased natural miscarriage rate at earlier gestations and to a slight increase in procedure-related loss. The culture failure rate and the inci-

---

Box 6.1   Indications for amniocentesis

Chromosomal analysis	Rarely required
Some single gene disorders	
PCR for viral infection (e.g. erythrovirus, cytomegalovirus)	—alphafetoprotein
	—acetylcholinesterase
Amnioreduction	
Amnioinfusion	

dence of fetal talipes are also higher when amniocentesis is performed at earlier gestations.

3. Now locate the placenta and assess the amniotic fluid, looking for the largest available pocket. It is preferable to avoid the placenta and to keep close to the midline. A puncture which is too lateral may encroach on uterine vessels or bowel. The inferior epigastric vessels run vertically behind the rectus sheath, and the midpoint between the anterior superior iliac spine and the umbilicus is a useful landmark on their course. A puncture-related injury is so rare that counselling relating to this is not required.

4. Sterile technique is essential. The abdominal skin should be cleansed with chlorhexidine, utilising sterile gel and a sterile transducer sleeve. Sterility can be enhanced by using a sterile drape such as a perineal towel (Fig. 6.3).

5. Repeat the scan specifically to visualise your target and align your transducer. Make sure your left to right orientation is correct. The transducer is marked at

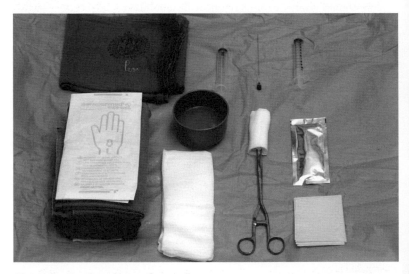

Fig. 6.3 Sterile technique for needling.

one end or you can orientate by simply indenting the abdominal wall with your finger and visualise simultaneously.

6. Under direct vision, insert a 90 mm long 22-gauge (G) needle (Fig. 6.4). The needle is of such small bore that local anaesthetic is not required. Remove the stylet and aspirate using 10 ml syringes. The first 1–2 ml are usually discarded because of possible maternal cell contamination which may grow on culture. 15–20 ml is sufficient for chromosomal analysis. If undertaking earlier amnio-centesis, the rule of thumb is 1 ml per week of gestation.

7. Ensure the sample is labelled correctly and transported immediately to the laboratory.

8. Prescribe anti-D 250 IU if the patient is Rhesus-negative.

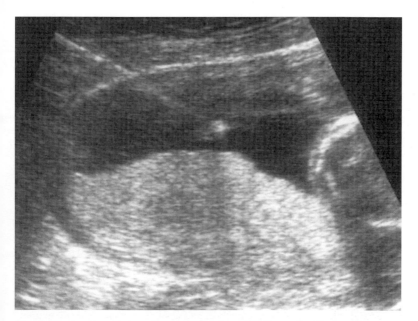

Fig. 6.4 *Amniocentesis – direct visualisation of 22G needle. The needle is inserted into the largest pool of amniotic fluid avoiding placenta, cord and fetus.*

Problems

1. *The obese patient.* The normal 90 mm needle may be too short. Measure the on-screen distance from the edge of your transducer to the centre of the liquor pool to give you an estimate of the depth. 125 and 180 mm needles are available. On occasions, it may be difficult to see the needle because of the attenuation caused by the subcutaneous fat.

2. *Anterior placenta.* If the placenta cannot be avoided, you will have to perform a transplacental tap. Do this away from the cord insertion and not too near the edge. The loss rate appears to be similar in skilled hands. The chances of a blood-stained tap may be slightly higher.

3. *Blood-stained tap.* The sample may be blood-stained from transplacental passage of the needle or, more commonly, if there has been previous vaginal bleeding arising from the placenta and passing into the amniotic fluid.

4. *Failed tap.* If you try twice and fail, ask someone else to do it, preferably after an interval of 1 week. Check where the needle tip is. It may have come up against the posterior uterine wall or the fetus, or it may have been inadvertently pulled back. If you find that it is in the correct place but there is still no fluid, it is most likely that the membranes have tented (Fig. 6.5). Replace the stylet and rotate the needle. If this fails, pushing the needle further towards the posterior wall may help. Failing this, abandon the procedure and try again in 1 week.

5. *Twins.* Before proceeding, you require to map the pregnancy, drawing in the case notes the position of each sac, the dividing membrane and the placental sites in relation to the maternal abdomen. Thus you will determine which twin is inferior and leading (twin 1) or superior (twin 2), left or right (Fig. 6.6). Label your specimen tubes and be sure to put the correct sample into the correct tube. The usual technique is to undertake two separate amniocenteses from each sac. Some operators inject indigo carmine into the first sac to ensure that it is not tapped again. Methylene blue is contraindicated, having been associated with intestinal atresia. However, careful mapping is normally sufficient. Others have described a single-needle approach, aspirating from one sac and then passing the needle through the septum. This can result in amniotic sac rupture and there is the risk of cross-contamination of amniotic fluid.

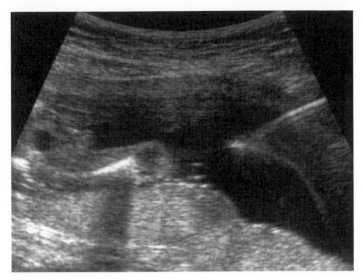

Fig. 6.5 *Tenting of the membranes seen. The needle was inserted further with a swift movement to ensure penetration into the amniotic fluid.*

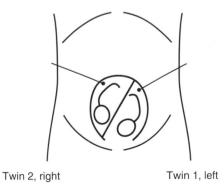

Twin 2, right   Twin 1, left

Fig. 6.6 *Map of amniocenteses showing needle insertion points and labelling to identify each twin.*

Checklist for amniocentesis

Counsel about procedure, miscarriage risk, culture failure, time to report
Scan for gestation, placental site, largest pool of amniotic fluid
Sterile technique
22G needle
Aspirate 15–20 ml amniotic fluid at 15 weeks
Label sample correctly
Rhesus status and 250 IU anti-D if appropriate

Points to remember

1. Align needle and transducer.
2. Practise on a fluid-filled model.
3. 30 supervised procedures for competence.
4. Risk of miscarriage 0.5–1%.
5. Risk of failed culture 1%.

Case Scenario (Fig. 6.7)

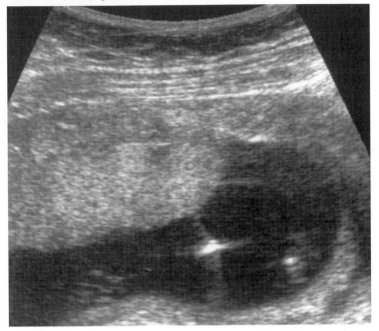

Incorrect insertion of needle through the edge of the placenta. It would have been preferable to take the clear approach from the opposite side avoiding the placenta. However, the amniotic fluid was not blood-stained and no complications resulted.

Chorion biopsy

Chorion biopsy, also known as chorion villus sampling (CVS), was introduced into obstetric practice in the mid-1980s, heralded as a first trimester test for determination of karyotype. Its advantages over second trimester amniocentesis were earlier diagnosis and, for affected pregnancies, early suction termination as opposed to a mid-trimester-induced labour after fetal movements had been experienced. It reached a peak in popularity by the late 1980s but demand declined because of the false-positive results associated with placental mosaicism (1%), the slightly higher reported risk of miscarriage (2%) compared to later amniocentesis (0.5–1%), the media attention given to the potential association with limb abnormalities, and the introduction of earlier amniocentesis and biochemical screening. The Royal College of Obstetricians and Gynaecologists recommend that CVS should only be undertaken after 10 completed weeks (10+0) to avoid the potential risk of limb malformations and it has been shown to be safer than early amniocentesis.

In the last 5 years, the demand for CVS has increased again. This is due to the advent of nuchal translucency and early biochemical screening and the ability to test the sample in 48 hours for trisomies using polymerase chain reaction (PCR). In addition, the loss rate in experienced hands is less than previously found (now 1%) and is safer than early amniocentesis and comparable to later amniocentesis.

In addition to karyotyping, the test is indicated in the detection of certain single gene disorders (Box 6.2).

Box 6.2 Indications for chorion villus sampling

Single gene disorders
—cystic fibrosis
—Huntington's disease
—muscular dystrophy
—sickle cell disease
—thalassaemia
—haemophilia
—metabolic disorders

Chromosomal
—maternal age
—increased nuchal translucency
—parental translocation

In early pregnancy the chorion appears homogeneous and surrounds the amniotic sac but by 10 weeks it has differentiated into the chorion frondosum (frond-like) and the chorion laeve (smooth). The chorion frondosum is called the placenta in later pregnancy (Fig. 4.3). The chorion frondosum is more accessible by transabdominal sampling if it is formed near the fundus of the uterus and by the transcervical route if it is formed low and posteriorly. Transabdominal needle aspiration is usually possible and is the more common approach because the pregnancy loss rate is slightly less; however, more skill is required to master this technique.

1. First, scan the uterus to ascertain the gestational age from crown–rump length (CRL) measurement and establish viability.

2. Check where the chorion frondosum has formed and ascertain your approach. It is best to hold the transducer centrally, in the longitudinal plane. A slightly distended bladder is helpful, but not too full since this will make access difficult.

3. If you choose the transabdominal approach, the same sterile precautions are required as for amniocentesis. An 18/21G needle combination is used. Many centres use a single needle but a smaller sample size will be obtained and, if inadequate, a second insertion is required. Draw up 10 ml 1% lidocaine, align your transducer and inject 1 ml of the local anaesthetic into the skin site using a fine needle. Replace the fine needle with a larger gauge and, using ultrasound guidance, inject the remains of your local anaesthetic into the rectus sheath, peritoneal surfaces and superficial myometrium. This is your opportunity to determine your final needle direction. Remove the needle and insert the 18G needle, following the same path. Significant pressure is sometimes required if the skin is tough. Follow the needle with your ultrasound imaging, having your intended target site in view. A rapid, forceful movement is required when penetrating the uterine wall and if this intention is not followed, the uterus will move posteriorly and you will miss your target site. A loss of resistance is experienced when the needle enters the chorion. Remove the stylet and insert the 21G needle with attached 20 ml syringe. The 21G needle is 2 cm longer when fully inserted and you must follow its penetration into the chorion. Now move it in and out, over this 2 cm length with suction applied on the syringe. A biopsy aspirator may be attached to aid the suction. Flush your sample into sterile transport medium. You normally require at least four aspirates to have enough tissue for culture, sometimes more depending on the test required.

4. If the chorion is not accessible by the transabdominal approach, then the choice is to wait 1 week or undertake a transcervical biopsy. With this route, it

is easier to have an assistant to perform the abdominal scan. Cleanse the perineal skin, insert a speculum to visualise the cervix. Take a cervical swab for culture and then clean with Savlon. With an anteverted uterus and the chorion sited posteriorly, it is usually fairly straightforward to insert the cannula correctly under direct vision. Attach a 20 ml syringe, apply suction and move the cannula gently to and fro for 1–2 cm, two to three times. On the last occasion, remove completely, maintaining suction throughout and then flush the specimen into culture medium. You may wish to place some culture medium in the syringe beforehand. One insertion is usually sufficient if placement is correct.

5. Give anti-D 250 IU if Rhesus-negative.

Checklist for chorion biopsy

Counsel patient
Scan for viability, gestation
Identify chorion frondosum
Visualise your needle path
18/21G needle combination
Rhesus status and 250 IU anti-D if appropriate

Points to remember

1. Undertake after 10 weeks.
2. Risk of miscarriage 1–2%.
3. Risk of mosaicism 1%.
4. Risk of failed culture 1%.

Case Scenario (Fig. 6.8)

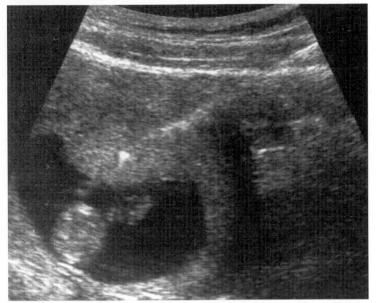

This transabdominal chorion biopsy was undertaken at 11 weeks for genetic studies to exclude Menkes' syndrome. The mother was a carrier for this rare X-linked disorder of copper metabolism. An 18/22G needle combination was used and the tip can be seen in the chorion frondosum. The fetal karyotype was 46XY and the maternal X chromosome did not carry the affected gene. The pregnancy progressed without complication thereafter.

Fetal blood sampling

Fetal blood sampling was also introduced into obstetric practice in the mid-1980s, virtually replacing fetoscopy overnight. Its main roles have been for rapid fetal karyotyping when a late diagnosis of fetal abnormality or intrauterine growth restriction (IUGR) has been made, for diagnosis of fetal genetic disorders, for intrauterine intravascular blood transfusion in cases of Rhesus and other blood group incompatibilities, and for the diagnosis of intrauterine infection. The indications are declining because of advances in molecular genetics with karyotype and infection being diagnosed quickly by polymerase chain reaction (PCR) on amniotic fluid samples. Most genetic disorders can now be diagnosed from chorion. Now, the main reason for accessing the fetal circulation via the umbilical vein is to determine haematocrit and transfuse if necessary. The earliest gestation is 18 weeks and the procedure obviously becomes easier as the vessels enlarge.

1. Perform a preliminary scan to assess the fetus and then look specifically for the placenta and cord insertion. Colour flow Doppler may help but it results in loss of resolution and thus is limited to identification of the insertion site. Aim to puncture the umbilical vein about 1 cm from the placental insertion – a transplacental approach is easiest. Other sites are free-floating cord, the umbilical cord insertion, the intrahepatic portion of umbilical vein or the fetal heart.

2. Employing sterile technique, visualise your local anaesthetic needle to judge direction to your target site and inject 5 ml 1% lidocaine down to the rectus sheath, peritoneum and uterine serosa. Employing the free-hand technique, use a 20G needle and advance your needle in the same direction so that it is close to your target vessel. A brisk intentional movement is required to penetrate the wall.

Box 6.3 Indications for fetal blood sampling

Blood group isoimmunisation
Unexplained hydrops
Alloimmune thrombocytopenia

3. Ask your assistant to remove the stylet and look for blood entering the chamber. Attach a syringe and take your sample. If there is no blood, check where the needle tip is sited. Rotating the needle may help, applying some suction on the syringe at the same time. Failing this, slight forward or backward motion may result in success.

4. Confirm that you are in the correct vessel by injecting 1 ml saline and visualising the flush on the screen or your laboratory can check by mean red cell volume or Kleihauer test.

5. Give 250 IU anti-D if Rhesus-negative and no antibodies.

Checklist for fetal blood sampling

Placenta, cord insertion
Colour flow Doppler
Visualise target site
20G needle
Confirm fetal blood
Rhesus status and 250 IU anti-D if appropriate

Points to remember

1. Earliest gestation is 18 weeks.
2. Main indication is fetal transfusion.

6.5

Intracardiac injection

Late termination for fetal abnormality

When late termination of pregnancy is being undertaken after 20 weeks' gestation, it is preferable on compassionate grounds for fetus, mother and staff that fetal death has been confirmed prior to delivery. Intracardiac injection of potassium chloride (KCl) will ensure this. The procedure, termed feticide, is similar to fetal blood sampling and relatively easier because of the larger structure.

1. Give sedation for both maternal and fetal benefit. There are different regimens: lorazepam, 4 mg orally 2 hours beforehand, with morphine 5 mg and prochlorperazine 12.5 mg intramuscularly 1 hour beforehand is effective.

2. Draw up 10 ml 10% KCl and make sure this is identified separately from your local anaesthetic.

3. Follow the technique as described for fetal blood sampling. Use local anaesthetic and align your 20G needle towards the fetal heart. It is easier if the fetus is supine. Once the needle is close to the fetus, a rapid movement is again required.

4. Confirm that the needle position is correct by aspirating fetal blood. You may wish to send this for chromosomal analysis or further investigations.

5. Inject 4–6 ml 10% KCl and asystole is virtually immediate if the needle position is correct.

6. Rest your transducer and after 5 minutes, confirm terminal bradycardia or asystole. Finally check 1–2 hours later.

Checklist for fetocide
Offer sedation 20G needle Confirm fetal blood 4–10 ml 10% KCl Check for terminal bradycardia Confirm asystole 1–2 hours later

Points to remember
1. Ensure correct placement of needle in fetal circulation before injecting KCl.
2. This is an unpleasant procedure for all concerned but alleviates maternal and neonatal suffering.

Multifetal reduction

Transabdominal intrathoracic injection of KCl may also be required for multifetal pregnancy reduction. The purpose of this is to reduce the risk of preterm delivery which is associated with triplet and higher-order pregnancies. The mean gestational age of delivery for triplets is 33 weeks and the perinatal mortality rate is around 80/1000 with an 80% risk of neonatal morbidity and a 10% risk of neurodevelopmental handicap. Fetal reduction to two would improve these statistics but the procedure is associated with risk of miscarriage which is 4% and doubles to 8% if reducing four to two and 12% if reducing five to two, the loss correlating with the initial and final numbers. Success rates improve with experience. The optimum timing appears to be 10–11 weeks by which time viability has been confirmed. If reduction is undertaken after this time, the risk of miscarriage or preterm delivery appears to increase. For this reason, if lethal abnormality is diagnosed in one twin, it is preferable not to undertake selective fetocide because the risk of preterm labour is higher than if the pregnancy were left alone.

1. First, locate the positions of the fetuses, check the number and confirm viability. Measure each CRL, look for any identifiable abnormality and determine chorionicity (see Ch. 2). If two fetuses share a chorion (monochorionic), a single fetus cannot be selected.

2. Determine which fetus is most accessible. Avoid the lower sac if possible.

3. Draw a map of the positions of each sac in relation to the maternal abdomen and clearly identify which selection has been made.

4. Follow the same needle-guided procedure as before, using a 20 or 22G, and aim for the fetal chest. The needle does not require to penetrate the heart. Injection of 1–2 ml 10% KCl is usually sufficient to create asystole within seconds.

5. Keep the needle in place for a couple of minutes and reconfirm that there is cessation of cardiac activity.

6. Repeat your scan the next day to make absolutely sure.

7. If reduction of more than one fetus is required, separate needle punctures are usually required, although sometimes one fetus may lie directly beneath another.

Checklist for multifetal reduction

Number, viability, CRL, chorionicity
Draw map of positions
Choose most accessible fetus
Recheck chorionicity
20 or 22G needle
Fetal chest
1–2 ml 10% KCl
Check next day
Rhesus status and 250 IU anti-D if appropriate

Points to remember

1. 10–11 weeks optimal.
2. If two fetuses share a chorion, it is inappropriate to select one.
3. Procedure reduces risk of preterm delivery.
4. 4% risk of miscarriage for reduction of triplets to twins.
5. Success rates improve with experience.

6.6

Other procedures

These include:

1. *Urine sampling.* In a minority of instances when there is an obstructive uropathy and progressive oligohydramnios, it may be appropriate to aspirate fetal urine from the bladder to measure the sodium and chloride content. If these are normal (sodium <100 mEq/l; chloride <90 mEq/l), then consideration can be given for insertion of a vesico-amniotic shunt. There are no large, long-term, follow-up studies of outcome.

2. *Amnioinfusion.* The instillation of fluid into the amniotic cavity when oligohydramnios is present has been used as a diagnostic procedure to establish the cause. This is rarely necessary.

3. *Amnioreduction.* Serial amnioreduction at around 10-day intervals has a place in the symptomatic relief of polyhydramnios and in the management of twin-to-twin transfusion syndrome. It is likely to reduce the risk of preterm delivery.

4. *Intraperitoneal infusion.* This may aid diagnosis of renal agenesis or differentiate a diaphragmatic hernia from cystic adenomatous lung malformation.

5. *Shunting.* This is when a pigtail catheter is inserted to permanently shunt a distended bladder or cystic lung lesion.

6. *Laser ablation.* This is used to ablate connecting vessels in monochorionic twin pregnancies.

We are now at the limits of *Obstetric Ultrasound Made Easy* and refer you to more weighty tomes if you need more information.

Case Scenario (Fig. 6.9 A, B)

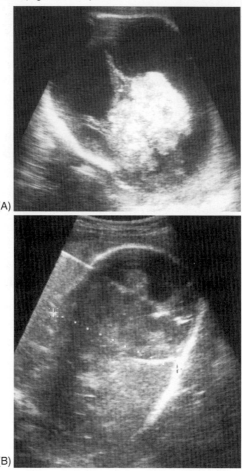

(A)

(B)

*Hydrocephaly had enlarged this fetal head such that the biparietal diameter was 13 cm. Porencephalic cysts were also evident **(A)**. The prognosis for the fetus was grim. Safe vaginal delivery was made possible following decompression and reduction in size of the head **(B)**.*

SECTION 2

Gynaecology

How to undertake a gynaecological scan

Preparing the patient and yourself

It is important to be aware of certain practicalities when undertaking a gynaecological ultrasound examination because a transvaginal scan will normally be required. Explain to the patient what the examination entails. Obtain verbal consent by asking the patient if she is happy with the explanation and willing for you to proceed. A chaperone should be present and preferably unrelated to the woman. This is important as the chaperone is a witness to what is happening and is also a source of support. Facilities should be available for the woman to change in privacy and comfort. She may need some guidance and help, particularly if elderly. A gown or sheet should be available to maintain dignity and the patient should not be left undressed for long. The procedure should be undertaken in a private setting, preferably in a room which can be locked to avoid unexpected intrusion.

Always maintain professionalism and avoid personal remarks relating to body appearance such as suntans, tattoos or piercing. Address the patient by her preferred name and avoid terms of endearment such as 'love', 'dear' or 'lass'. Your examination should be skilful and gentle. You should be alert to any discomfort or pain experienced by the patient. Explain to the patient what you are doing and what is being seen on the screen. If the woman becomes distressed, ask if she wishes you to pause or stop the examination.

Checklist
Explanation of procedure
Verbal consent
Chaperone
Changing facility
Maintain professional approach
Be skilful and gentle

You require to know the indication for the gynaecological scan and it is essential to take a relevant clinical history beforehand. If the scan has been requested by another clinician, a completed (or incomplete!) request form should be available. It is worth going over this with the patient. Important points to take into account are the woman's age; menstrual history with date of last menstrual period (LMP); any abdominal or pelvic pain; medication, particularly hormonal; previous gynaecological history. You may find a checklist helpful.

Checklist for gynaecological history

History of presenting complaint
Menstrual history with date of LMP
Menstrual cycle (length, regularity, duration of period, flow – normal, scanty, heavy)
Abnormal bleeding (intermenstrual, postcoital, postmenopausal)
Pain (dysmenorrhoea, dyspareunia, abdominal)
Vaginal discharge
Method of contraception
Other hormonal treatment (assisted reproduction, hormone replacement, progestogens, tamoxifen)
Previous gynaecological problems and operations
Previous pregnancies (if any)

The patient is likely to have had a gynaecological examination already and you should check the findings. A knowledge of the basic anatomy of the pelvic organs is essential (Fig. 7.1). With a combination of transabdominal and transvaginal scanning, you should be able to visualise the bladder, uterus and ovaries. If a lower abdominal or pelvic mass is suspected, it is better to undertake a transabdominal

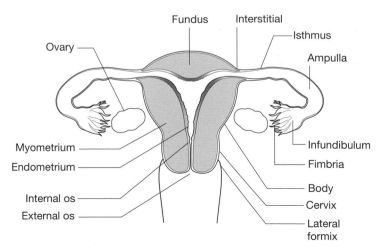

Fig. 7.1 *The anatomy of the pelvic organs.*

scan first. The focal range of the transvaginal transducer is approximately 8–10 cm which means that any structure outwith this range will be missed. A very enlarged uterus or ovarian cyst may rise out of the pelvis and will not be visualised by a transvaginal scan. You will miss it unless you do a transabdominal scan!

The transabdominal scan

It is essential that the bladder is full when scanning the pelvis transabdominally. This is not normally required for a transvaginal scan. A full bladder provides an acoustic window through which the pelvic structures can be visualised. There are a variety of transabdominal transducers (Fig. 1.2) and a 3.5 MHz transducer is suitable. It is important to have a structured approach to your scan.

1. Having checked the indication for the scan and obtained verbal consent, invite the woman to lie on a suitable couch. She should then be asked to re-arrange her clothes to expose her lower abdomen. Protective tissue paper should be placed to cover her lower garments and at the same time ensure that the abdomen is exposed immediately above the symphysis pubis.

2. Having applied ultrasound gel, place the transducer longitudinally above the symphysis pubis to identify the bladder. Through this it will be possible to visualise the pelvic organs.

3. Locate the uterus. This provides a central landmark for scanning the pelvis. If the woman has had a hysterectomy then the full bladder is used as the central pelvic landmark.

4. Assess the uterine size. You may wish to measure the uterus and there are normal values for the different phases of women's life (see Ch. 8). As you gain experience, you will be able to recognise normal size or not.

5. Describe the position of the uterus, and whether it is anteverted or retroverted (Fig. 7.2A); see also Figure 8.3.

6. Move the transducer from side to side in the longitudinal plane to visualise the whole of the myometrium. It is also worthwhile rotating the transducer to obtain transverse views of the myometrium (Fig. 7.2B). Look for areas of increased echogenicity or calcification; these may indicate fibroids and are described further in Chapter 8.

7. Move the transducer inferiorly in the longitudinal plane to visualise the cervix which is located at the lower pole of the uterus. It is more easily seen transvaginally but it is important to locate because occasionally a cervical polyp or fibroid may be seen.

8. Locate the endometrium in the centre of the uterus and it is best visualised in the longitudinal plane. The endometrium varies in appearance according to

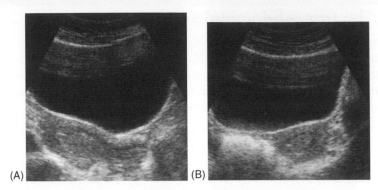

Fig. 7.2 *Transabdominal scan showing:* **(A)** *sagittal section of normal anteverted uterus and cervix;* **(B)** *transverse section of normal uterus.*

hormonal influences or pathology and its thickness is measured when there is a clinical indication (see Ch. 8).

9. Now move the transducer laterally in the transverse plane to visualise the adnexa. You will not require much lateral movement if the bladder is full (Fig. 7.3). The structures of interest are the fallopian tubes and ovaries. The fallopian tubes tend *not* to be visualised unless they are filled with fluid (hydrosalpinx) or pus (pyosalpinx). Ovaries are most easily seen in women of reproductive age, their follicles making them identifiable. They are normally found medial to the iliac vessels but they can be located in a variety of positions ranging from the pouch of Douglas to the pelvic side wall. In postmenopausal women it is often not possible to visualise them. If you are having difficulty locating the ovaries, try turning the transducer laterally, placing the uterus in the centre of the image, and then look to the lateral aspect of the transducer and it may then be possible to locate them. The ovarian appearance also changes with hormonal influence and pathology; these issues will be discussed further in Chapter 9. Once the ovaries have been visualised, record any abnormal location, describe their appearance and measure them. *It is much easier to see ovaries with transvaginal ultrasound.*

10. There are some pitfalls to be aware of. For example, bowel can mimic ovaries or dilated fallopian tube in appearance and you can differentiate by holding the transducer still over the structure; if it is bowel then after a few seconds

you will see peristalsis. Vessels can mimic follicles and by rotating your transducer by 90 degrees the follicle may then become 'tube like' and therefore most likely to be a vessel. If you have colour Doppler, flow can be identified in a suspected vessel.

11. Posterior to the uterus lies the pouch of Douglas or recto-uterine fossa. Using transabdominal ultrasound it will not be seen unless it contains fluid. A small amount of fluid is normal but an excessive echo-free pool is abnormal in keeping with ascites or blood.

Unless excellent views of the pelvis are obtained with transabdominal ultrasound, or there was a contraindication to using transvaginal ultrasound (see Section 7.3), then transvaginal ultrasound should be undertaken. Both techniques complement one another.

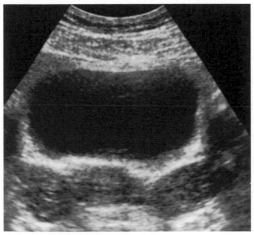

Fig. 7.3 *Transabdominal scan showing both ovaries on each side of the uterus.*

The transvaginal scan

Transvaginal ultrasound has the advantage that the structures lying proximal to the transducer will be clearly visualised. Most transvaginal transducers are high frequency probes (5–7.5 MHz) – the higher the frequency the better the resolution but the lower the penetration. From the tip of the probe, structures can be visualised up to 10 cm. Structures beyond this distance will be missed.

Orientation and transducer movement to locate the uterus and ovaries

Although transvaginal ultrasound gives better views of the structures within the pelvis, there is less scope to manoeuvre the probe due to the limited space within the vagina. You should hold the transducer with the right hand and your thumb should be placed uppermost. Most probes have a small dimple in the handle of the probe to place your thumb. This helps greatly with orientation of the transducer. There are a variety of different possible movements of the vaginal probe and you should familiarise yourself with these to ensure a logical approach to your technique.

1. **Sliding** (Fig. 7.4A)

This is the first movement made when the probe is inserted into and along the length of the vagina. The direction of the vagina is downwards and backwards. It is with this movement that the landmark for the pelvis, the uterus, is often located. However, a little rocking movement is usually required.

2. **Rocking** (Fig. 7.4B)

Rocking is movement of the transducer in the anteroposterior plane. Once the transducer is inserted, gently move the probe handle up and down until the uterus comes into the field of vision. When the uterus is anteverted, the tip of the probe will normally stop in the posterior fornix (Fig. 7.2A). By gently moving the probe handle upwards the uterus should come into view. Conversely, if the uterus is retroverted, the probe naturally rests in the anterior fornix of the vagina and gentle movement of the probe downwards will help locate the uterus. When you begin the scan you frequently do not know the position of the uterus and the combination of sliding and rocking is essential to locate the uterus.

3. Panning (Fig. 7.4C)

Once the uterus has been located then the next step is to visualise the adnexa and ovaries and panning is necessary for this. This is movement in the horizontal plane. Having obtained a transverse image of the uterus, move the probe handle to the right to visualise the right adnexum. Sometimes the ovaries will be visualised with this movement alone, but generally the probe has to be rotated.

4. Rotating (Fig. 7.4D)

This describes the circular movements with the handle of the probe. If the transducer is rotated 90 degrees from the longitudinal (sagittal), then this gives a transverse (horizontal) view. So by panning to the right and rotating the probe about 45 degrees outwards the iliac vessels should be visualised. The ovaries are generally found medial to these vessels. It is easy to see the ovaries in a premenopausal woman because they contain numerous follicles.

Once the right ovary has been located, rotate the transducer back to the neutral position and pan to the left to visualise the left adnexum. The same steps of panning and rotation should be undertaken to visualise the left internal iliac vessels and left ovary. The left ovary is less easy to identify because of shadowing from the sigmoid colon. The ovaries are not always located in the expected places and can be found in the pouch of Douglas or high up in the pelvic side wall. As stated previously it may not always be possible to visualise the ovaries in postmenopausal women, even using transvaginal ultrasound.

Checklist for transvaginal probe movements

Sliding – insertion into the vagina downwards and backwards
Rocking – up and down movement in the anteroposterior plane
Panning – horizontal movement from left to right
Rotating – circular movement of 90 degrees from longitudinal to transverse view

---

Approach to the transvaginal scan

1. Check the history and reason for the scan. Check that there are no contraindications (see Box 7.1), explain what the examination entails and obtain verbal consent. Comparing the procedure to an internal examination gives most women an idea of what to expect.

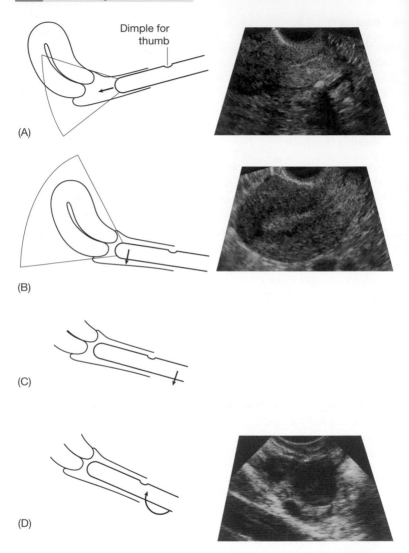

Fig. 7.4 Orientation and transducer movements. *(A)* Sliding to locate the uterus. *(B)* Rocking to visualise the whole uterus. *(C)* Panning to the adnexum. *(D)* Rotating to visualise the iliac vessels and ovary.

2. Arrange for the patient to empty her bladder, remove her underwear (and tampon if appropriate) and drape herself with a gown or sheet. If the woman has had a hysterectomy or is postmenopausal then it is useful to keep some urine in the bladder as a useful landmark for orientation in the pelvis.

3. Invite the woman to lie on a suitable couch. There are a variety of options for positioning the patient. She may lie on a couch with a pillow placed under her buttocks to elevate the pelvis (Fig. 7.5A), she may lie on a lithotomy couch (Fig. 7.5B) or she may have her buttocks resting at the end of the bed with her feet supported by a chair (Fig. 7.5C).

4. Wear disposable gloves. Apply coupling gel to the tip of the probe and cover it with a condom. The condom should be pulled tightly over the tip of the probe to avoid 'air trapping'. Then apply gel to the tip of the covered probe.

5. Hold the probe in your right hand and inform the patient that you are about to pass it. You may require to part the labia with your left hand. Gently insert the probe, using the minimum of force and remembering that the direction of the vagina is downwards and backwards. If you have used your left hand to part the labia, the glove should be removed so that the controls on the ultrasound machine can be operated.

6. Evaluate the uterus, ovaries and adnexa as previously described.

7. An explanation about the different movements should be given to the patient and when the examination is finished the probe should be withdrawn gently.

8. Assist the patient off the couch, maintaining her dignity throughout.

Box 7.1 Contraindications to transvaginal imaging

Children
Virgo intacta
Some elderly postmenopausal women
Large mass
Psychosexual disorder

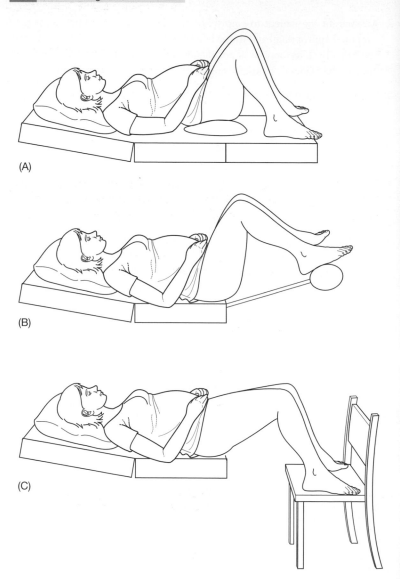

Fig. 7.5 *Positioning of the patient for transvaginal ultrasound scan:* **(A)** *pillow under buttocks;* **(B)** *lithotomy poles;* **(C)** *chair.*

Reporting your findings

It is useful to have standard request and reporting forms which can be computerised for audit purposes. An example which incorporates both and can be easily computerised is shown in Box 7.2. The advantage of a standard request form is that it helps to ensure that the referring clinician does not omit relevant clinical details. The reporting form should have a simple structured layout. If the pelvis is normal then only ticks are required. It is important to have a comments box for further elaboration of your findings or if something unusual is detected.

Box 7.2 Example of structured gynaecological ultrasound request and report form

Parity   LMP

Symptoms		*Clinical information*	
RIF pain	☐	Vaginal exam not possible	☐
LIF pain	☐	Normal findings	☐
Central pain	☐	Pelvic inflammatory disease	☐
Dysmenorrhoea	☐	Fibroid	☐
Dyspareunia	☐	Right adnexal mass	☐
Postmenopausal bleeding	☐	Left adnexal mass	☐
Amenorrhoea	☐	PCO suspected	☐
Oligomenorrhoea	☐	Latex allergy	☐
Menorrhagia	☐		
Intermenstrual bleeding	☐		

Additional clinical comments e.g. previous surgery:

Referring clinician: Grade:

Report
Date:

Uterus		*Ovaries*	R	L
Normal	☐	Normal	☐	☐
Absent	☐	Absent	☐	☐
Fibroids	☐	Not demonstrated	☐	☐
Size: cm × cm × cm		Cyst	☐	☐
Endometrial thickness mm		Size: cm × cm × cm		
		Free fluid: present/absent		

Further comments:

Describe further any abnormalities (fibroids, ovarian cysts):

Name and designation:

Checklist for gynaecological scan

Uterine size, position
Myometrium
Cervix
Endometrium
Ovaries
Other adnexal abnormalities

Points to remember

1. Transabdominal and transvaginal scanning complement one another.
2. Transvaginal probes have higher frequencies than transabdominal probes.
3. Transvaginal probes have a maximum field of vision of 8–10 cm.

The uterus

Physiological changes in the endometrium during the menstrual cycle

An understanding of the physiological changes seen in the endometrium during the menstrual cycle is necessary for the correct interpretation of your ultrasonic findings (Fig. 8.1). The average length of the menstrual cycle is 28 days and the first day of the menstrual period is referred to as day 1 of the cycle. During the menstrual cycle sequential changes take place in the ovaries and endometrium; those seen in the ovary are described in Chapter 9.

In the first half of the cycle, the changes which occur in the endometrium are due to the influence of oestrogen. This is produced by the cells in the ovarian follicle. It causes the endometrium to thicken and proliferate. This is consequently called the follicular or proliferative phase of the menstrual cycle. In the second half of the cycle, the changes are due to the influence of oestrogen and progesterone which are produced by the cells in the corpus luteum. The endometrium thickens further, becoming spongy. The endometrial glands enlarge and start to secrete nutrients, becoming ready to receive and nourish a possible fertilised ovum. This is consequently called the luteal or secretory phase of the cycle.

If fertilisation fails to occur, the corpus luteum degenerates. Oestrogen and progesterone production decreases and the endometrium is no longer supported. Menstruation then occurs with the shedding of the endometrium.

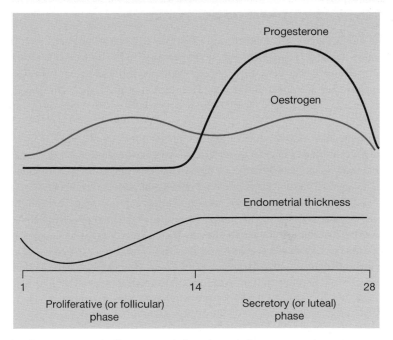

Fig. 8.1 *Hormonal influences and physiological changes to endometrium during the menstrual cycle.*

8.2

Normal uterine appearance

The uterus is the main solid structure that you will see in the pelvis on ultrasound scanning. The uterus normally lies posterior to the sonolucent bladder in the midline but may be pushed laterally by a very full bladder or pathology. It obviously lies anterior to the rectum. The position of the uterus is described as anteverted when it tilts forwards and retroverted when it tilts backwards (Fig. 8.2).

In a woman of reproductive age, the uterus normally measures 6–8 cm in length from fundus to external cervical os. The maximum transverse measurement is 5 cm and anteroposterior 4 cm. The measurements are 1–2 cm more in parous women and 1–2 cm less before puberty and after the menopause.

The uterine wall has a serosal surface which is the visceral peritoneum covering the muscularis or myometrium. The outline of the uterus is identified from the reflective echoes of the serosal surface. The myometrium has a homogeneous appearance with low level echoes and the echo-dense line of the endometrium confirms that the visualised structure is the uterus. The direction of the endometrial echo will inform you if the position is anteverted or retroverted (Fig. 8.3).

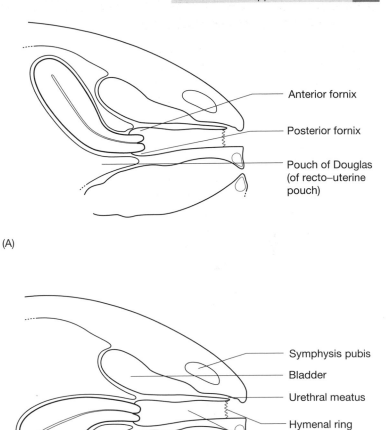

(A)

(B)

Fig. 8.2 *Anatomical positions of the uterus. (A = anteverted; B =retroverted.)*

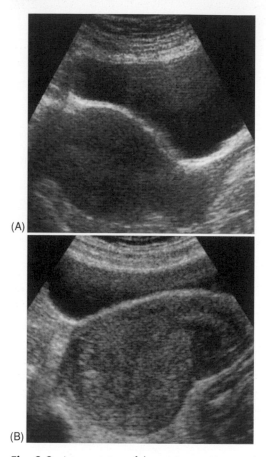

Fig. 8.3 Interpretation of the uterine position on ultrasound imaging. **(A)** Anteverted uterus. **(B)** Retroverted uterus.

8.3

Normal endometrial appearance

The endometrium is easy to differentiate from the myometrium, being more echogenic than the myometrium with an echo-poor layer separating them (Fig. 8.4). The anatomical basis for this echo-poor layer is not clear. It is more prominent after ovulation and before menstruation.

With the advent of transvaginal ultrasound, it has become possible to evaluate the physiological and pathological changes of the endometrium. To do this, you need to master the standard technique for measuring endometrial thickness.

1. Check the clinical indication for the ultrasound examination and take a menstrual history, noting the date of the last menstrual period.

2. Prepare the equipment, position the patient and insert the probe as previously described (see Ch. 7).

3. Locate the uterus and identify the echo-bright homogeneous endometrial echo.

4. Rotate the transducer until you obtain a sagittal view of the uterus and visualise the anterior and posterior endometrial layers and the echogenic line which signifies their interface.

5. Locate the area of endometrium of maximum thickness and place one cursor on the outer aspect of one layer and the second cursor on the outer aspect of the other layer, perpendicular to the long axis of the uterine cavity. Now record the measurement which is termed the 'endometrial thickness' incorporating both layers of endometrium (Fig. 8.4).

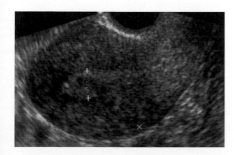

Fig. 8.4 Sagittal view of the uterus showing the endometrium and measurement of endometrial thickness.

6. If there is fluid in the endometrial cavity then each layer must be measured separately and the sum of both taken for the endometrial thickness value (Fig. 8.5). A small amount of fluid within the endometrial cavity may be seen as a normal finding. An excessive amount may be due to blood (haematometra) (Fig. 8.6) or pus (pyometra).

Fig. 8.5 *Sagittal view of the uterus showing measurement of the endometrial thickness when there is fluid in the endometrial cavity. The superior measurement was 1 mm and the inferior 0.7 mm, giving an endometrial thickness measurement of 1.7 mm.*

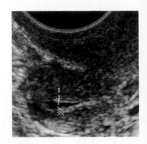

Case Scenario (Fig. 8.6)

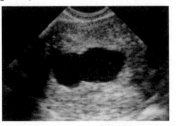

This 37-year-old patient attended with cyclical lower abdominal pain. She had had microwave endometrial ablation 9 months previously and this had obviously resulted in cervical stenosis with blood being trapped within the uterine cavity. Cervical dilatation gave immediate relief.

The endometrial thickness and appearance change during different phases of the menstrual cycle (Fig. 8.7). After menstruation a fine intracavity line is seen with no endometrial layer visualised. During the proliferative phase the endometrium may measure 2–4 mm with an echo-poor appearance. After ovulation an echo-poor halo is seen between the endometrium and myometrium. During the secretory phase the endometrium increases to 5–6 mm and even up to 14 mm is considered normal. There may be a trace of endometrial fluid at the time of ovulation and during menstruation. It is not always necessary to measure endometrial thickness routinely unless there is a clinical indication (e.g. postmenopausal bleeding).

After the menopause the uterus becomes significantly smaller and the endometrium is seen as a very thin line and virtually disappears (Fig. 8.8). In women who experience postmenopausal bleeding (PMB), an endometrial thickness measurement is required. It has been shown that the thicker the endometrium, the greater is the likelihood of endometrial cancer. There is some debate as to the exact cut-off value but is generally accepted that a measurement of 4 mm or more warrants an endometrial biopsy unless the woman is taking exogenous hormones (see below).

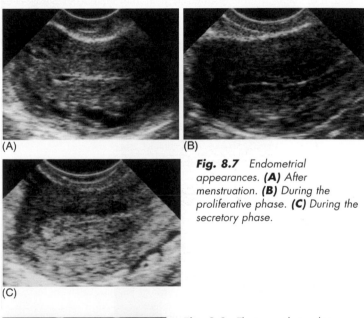

(A)

(B)

Fig. 8.7 *Endometrial appearances. (A) After menstruation. (B) During the proliferative phase. (C) During the secretory phase.*

(C)

Fig. 8.8 *The normal atrophic postmenopausal uterus with thin endometrial echo.*

Abnormal endometrial appearance

Endometrial polyps

Endometrial polyps are single pedunculated benign tumours found within the endometrial cavity. Histologically they are composed of hyperplastic endometrium, usually non-functional. The woman may be asymptomatic or present with abnormal bleeding, usually intermenstrual or postmenopausal. Ultrasonically, polyps are seen within the endometrial cavity as hyperechoic structures with small cystic areas (Fig. 8.9). They are often delineated by intra-cavity fluid. It can be difficult to distinguish them from submucous fibroids but these tend to be more hypoechoic (Fig. 8.10). It can also be difficult to differentiate

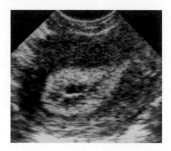

Fig. 8.9 *Endometrial polyp showing hyperechoic appearance with small cystic areas.*

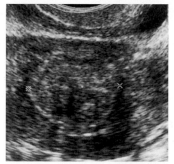

Fig. 8.10 *Intrauterine fibroid in a postmenopausal patient.*

between endometrial thickening and an endometrial polyp. This can be clarified by hysterosonography.

1. Fill a 10 ml syringe with sterile saline.

2. Insert a bivalve speculum into the vagina and locate the cervix.

3. Cleanse the cervix with a swab on a sponge-holding forceps.

4. Pass a fine plastic cannula 1–2 cm through the cervix to the approximate level of the internal os.

5. Remove the speculum.

6. Attach the syringe and inject slowly the sterile saline under ultrasound guidance until the endometrial cavity is outlined by the fluid; 2–3 ml are usually sufficient.

7. Inspect the outline of the endometrial cavity and any polyp should be clearly delineated.

The final diagnosis is usually made histologically following hysteroscopic resection.

Endometrial cancer

Endometrial cancer is the most common form of gynaecological cancer, predominantly occurring after the menopause when the patient presents with postmenopausal bleeding. In premenopausal women there may be a history of irregular menstrual loss or intermenstrual bleeding. Fortunately, the tumour tends to be slow growing and is usually confined to the uterus at the time of diagnosis. Infiltration into the broad ligaments and pelvic side walls occurs relatively late. The ultrasonic appearances of endometrial cancer can be variable but certain characteristics should be remembered. The endometrial thickness is increased (see below) and often has irregular margins. There is also increased echogenicity and there may be fluid in the cavity (Fig. 8.11). Excessive fluid in the uterine cavity may be due to blood (haematometra) or pus (pyometra). There may be evidence of invasion into the myometrium. Histological confirmation from endometrial biopsy is always required and abnormal ultrasound appearances will alert the clinician to investigate further.

Fig. 8.11 *Characteristic ultrasonic appearance of endometrial carcinoma with increased thickness and echogenicity, irregular margins and a small amount of intrauterine fluid.*

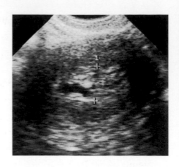

Exogenous hormones

Any medications which have oestrogenic or progestational effects will affect the endometrium.

1. The oral contraceptive pill causes endometrial hypoplasia and a characteristic single hyperechoic line is seen (Fig. 8.12). The endometrium is shed cyclically during the pill-free phase and so this finding is usually coincidental and does not have pathological consequences.

2. Hormone replacement therapy (HRT) is widely used to alleviate the peri-menopausal symptoms of hot flushes and mood swings. It may be used long term in a few patients who are at risk of osteoporosis. Long-term HRT has

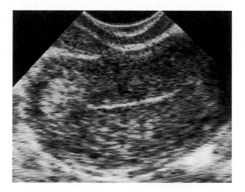

Fig. 8.12 *Single hyperechoic line seen in a patient who had been taking oral contraception for 6 months. Did you notice the small fibroid at the fundus?*

diminished considerably since the cardioprotective effect was found to be absent and the risks of breast and uterine cancer increased. There are various forms of HRT. Some are given as cyclical (or sequential) combined oestrogen and progesterone regimens inducing scheduled bleeding in most users. These cause thickening of the endometrium. Others are given as continuous combined when amenorrhoea results but there may be spotting or bleeding during the first year. These cause endometrial atrophy as does tibolone, another preparation which has combined oestrogen and progesterone properties.

The SIGN guideline on 'Investigation of postmenopausal bleeding' recommends an endometrial thickness of 3 mm or less to exclude endometrial cancer in women with PMB who have never used HRT or any HRT for at least a year or are using combined continuous HRT (SIGN 2002). This gives a post-test probability of cancer of 0.7%. An endometrial thickness of 5 mm or less is the recommended cut-off in women using (or having used in the preceding year) cyclical HRT. It is probably best to measure the endometrial thickness during the first half of the cycle. The post-test probability of cancer is 0.2%.

3. Tamoxifen is taken continuously for a period of time by patients who have had breast cancer. It is an anti-oestrogen binding to oestrogen receptors. Its effects on the endometrium vary and it may cause atrophy, polyps, hyperplasia and cancer. Patients on tamoxifen have an increased risk of up to six times of developing cancer and may be referred for endometrial thickness measurement if they have had abnormal vaginal bleeding. However, the diagnostic accuracy of ultrasound is not good because tamoxifen causes such varying effects on the endometrium. Hysteroscopy and endometrial biopsy are necessary for diagnosis (Fig. 8.13).

Case Scenario (Fig. 8.13)

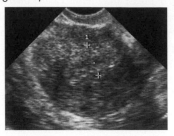

This 52-year-old patient presented with postmenopausal bleeding having been on tamoxifen for 3 years because of a previous breast cancer. The endometrial thickness measurement was 17 mm. She was referred for hysteroscopy and endometrial biopsy. The histology was reported as benign.

Remember that oestrogen-secreting ovarian tumours can also cause endometrial hyperplasia and you also need to check the ovaries.

Checklist for endometrial thickness measurement

Check clinical indication
Obtain a sagittal section of the uterus
Measure the maximum thickness perpendicular to the long axis of the uterus
Check the ovaries

Points to remember

1. Endometrial thickness is 2–4 mm in the proliferative phase and 5–14 mm in the secretory phase.
2. An endometrial thickness of 4 mm or more in a postmenopausal patient warrants an endometrial biopsy unless exogenous hormones are being taken.
3. An endometrial thickness of 3 mm or less excludes endometrial cancer with a post-test probability of cancer of 0.7%.

Abnormal myometrial appearance

Congenital abnormality of the uterus

Congenital uterine abnormalities are usually a coincidental finding but may be associated with infertility, recurrent miscarriage or preterm labour. The outline of the uterus may appear abnormal and there may be more than one complete or incomplete endometrial cavity (Fig. 8.14). The different abnormalities (described in Ch. 2, Fig. 2.37) result from abnormal fusion of the paramesonephric or müllerian ducts which form the uterus and proximal two-thirds of the vagina during embryogenesis. Magnetic resonance imaging can confirm and give a more detailed outline. 3-Dimensional ultrasound also appears promising. Be aware that if there is a congenital uterine abnormality, there may also be a renal abnormality because the paramesonephric ducts contribute to both systems.

Fibroids

Fibroids are benign tumours of the smooth muscle of the myometrium and they also have a variable proliferation of fibrous connective tissue. They tend to be spherical in shape and have a false capsule of compressed tissue. They are hard in consistency and their cut surface is white. Pathologists correctly identify them as myomas, fibromyomas, leiomyomas or fibroleiomyomas, but fibroids is the term most widely used.

Fibroids are frequently multiple and may grow to a very large size. They are located within the myometrium (intramural), under the serous surface of the uterus (subserosal) or under the endometrium (submucosal). Further descriptive

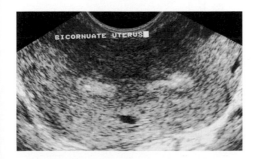

Fig. 8.14 *Two separate endometrial cavities at the fundus of a single uterus. The findings were in keeping with a bicornuate uterus.*

terminology is used depending on their location (Fig. 8.15). They are most commonly seen as intramural fibroids in asymptomatic women. They may arise at any time in a woman of reproductive age, most commonly causing symptoms after the age of 40. They are dependent on oestrogens for their growth and therefore tend to decrease in size after the menopause.

The symptoms that the woman experiences vary according to the site of the fibroid. This can vary from no symptoms, the feeling of a painless pelvic mass, intermenstrual bleeding or menorrhagia.

The submucosal group are those most commonly associated with clinical symptoms such as menorrhagia. Subserosal fibroids may be pedunculated and attached to a stalk, lying some distance from the uterus. They may undergo torsion and necrosis and the woman may present with pain. Submucosal fibroids may herniate into the vagina or cervix causing intermenstrual, postcoital bleeding or vaginal discharge.

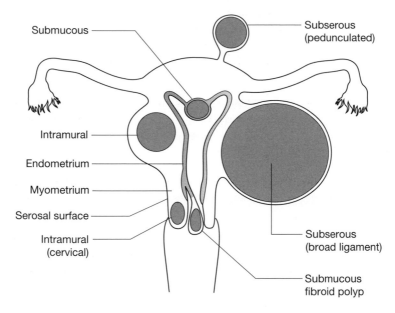

Fig. 8.15 *Potential sites of fibroid formation.*

The ultrasonic appearance of fibroids depends on the mix of smooth muscle and fibrous tissue. They may be hypo- or hyperechoic. They tend to have a homogeneous appearance unless they have undergone central degenerative change. They tend to be avascular, but the surrounding pseudocapsule is very vascular.

There are some tips on technique which may help.

1. Start your examination by performing a transabdominal scan. You may be able to identify fibroids within the uterus. A large fibroid may be outwith the pelvis and will be missed if you undertake a transvaginal scan only. The focal range of a transvaginal probe is usually a maximum of 10 cm.

2. If necessary, perform a transvaginal ultrasound examination and locate the uterus. Fibroids will be identified as roughly spherical structures of different echogenicity compared to the surrounding myometrium.

3. Define the location of the fibroid within uterus and measure in three dimensions (Fig. 8.16). The echogenicity of the fibroid should be noted, as cystic areas within the fibroid may suggest 'red degeneration' of the fibroid. If there are numerous fibroids it is clinically satisfactory to record that there is a fibroid uterus with multiple fibroids and to describe the location and dimensions of larger ones.

4. Ensure that the suspected fibroid mass is contained within the myometrium and continuous with the uterus. This will confirm that it is uterine in origin and not ovarian.

5. Identify the ovaries separately.

6. If you are fortunate to have good colour Doppler you can check to see that there will be little blood flow within the fibroid and ample blood flow in the pseudocapsule.

7. If there is a large broad ligament fibroid, it may be impossible for you to differentiate this from an ovarian cyst. Referral for magnetic resonance imaging may be necessary if the gynaecologist is concerned that the mass is an ovarian tumour.

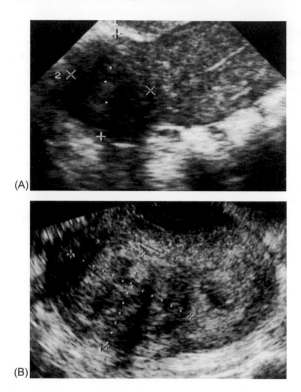

Fig. 8.16 **(A)** *30 × 23 × 25 mm echo-poor subserous fibroid seen on transvaginal scan in a postmenopausal patient.* **(B)** *37 × 48 × 45 mm circumscribed intramural fibroid in a 45-year-old woman presenting with menorrhagia.*

Checklist for suspected fibroids

Perform a transabdominal scan first. A transvaginal scan may not be necessary
Describe the location and 3-dimensional measurements
Check that fibroids are contiguous with the uterus and identify ovaries separately

---

Adenomyosis

Adenomyosis is when ectopic endometrial glands and stroma are found in the myometrium. Therefore it is a type of endometriosis but is more common in parous women presenting with menorrhagia and secondary dysmenorrhoea in their 40s. Endometriosis is more common in younger, nulliparous women. Adenomyosis is usually diagnosed after hysterectomy when it is detected histologically.

On ultrasound examination the uterus may appear entirely normal. It will be slightly enlarged but this is a normal finding in parous patients. Adenomatous lesions tend to be only 1–2 mm in size, when they are seen as small cystic areas within the myometrium; rarely they reach 1–2 cm in size, when ultrasonically they appear similar to fibroids.

Intrauterine contraceptive devices

There are two major forms of intrauterine contraceptive device (IUCD) in present use, one copper bearing and the other hormone releasing. Both are used for contraceptive purposes but the hormone-releasing variety is also used to treat menorrhagia by suppressing endometrial growth. The Mirena intrauterine system is the only hormone-releasing type in use in the UK. It is coated with the progestogen, levonorgestrel, which is slowly released.

The intrauterine presence of an IUCD is normally confirmed by the thread of the coil protruding through the cervix. If the thread is not seen or felt or a complication occurs (see Box 8.1), an ultrasound scan is useful to confirm that the IUCD is still within the uterine cavity. Sometimes the thread retracts into the cervical canal or falls off. Occasionally the IUCD may be expelled without the patient being aware or it may migrate out of the uterus into the peritoneal cavity and even into the pleural cavity.

1. If the patient has a full bladder, you may be able to visualise the uterine cavity clearly. If not, then a transvaginal scan is better.

2. If you see the IUCD within the uterine cavity, check that it is located centrally in both sagittal and coronal planes. Occasionally, it may be partially embedded in the uterine wall. The arms of IUCDs are not usually seen. The copper-containing coils are highly reflective and you will see acoustic shadowing (Fig. 8.17A). The Mirena coil is less echogenic and the ends are more obvious (Fig. 8.17B).

3. When you cannot see the IUCD within the uterine cavity then an abdominal X-ray will be required. All IUCDs are radio-opaque.

Box 8.1 Complications of IUCD requiring ultrasound assessment

Thread not seen or felt
Pelvic inflammatory disease
Pregnancy (see Ch. 2)
Suspected perforation at insertion

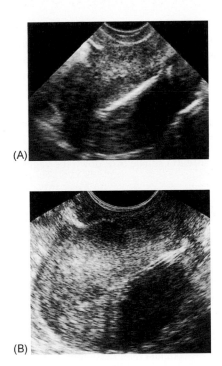

(A)

(B)

Fig. 8.17 (A) *Highly reflective Copper-T intrauterine contraceptive device seen within the uterine cavity.* **(B)** *The more echo-poor appearance of a Mirena intrauterine contraceptive device.*

The cervix

It is often difficult to visualise the cervix transabdominally. A full bladder is required and false elongation occurs. It is easier to visualise the cervix transvaginally and you should adhere to the following steps (assuming the uterus is anteverted):

1. Slide the transducer into the posterior fornix.

2. Gently rock the transducer by moving the handle downwards. This means the tip of the probe will move upwards bringing the uterus into view.

3. Slowly slide the transducer handle back down the vagina and the cervix will come into view.

Nabothian follicles

Nabothian follicles (or cysts) are retention cysts within the cervical glandular epithelium and are of no clinical significance. They appear as coincidental single or multiple echolucent, 0.5–1 cm circular structures (Fig. 8.18). They are frequently seen and should not be confused with an early gestational sac, especially one which may be lying in the cervical canal.

Cervical fibroid

Cervical fibroids are less common than those found in the body of the uterus. They are seen as echo-dense homogenous structures in the lower part of the

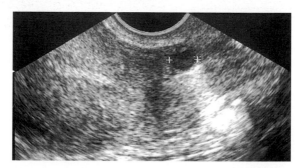

Fig. 8.18 9 mm Nabothian follicle seen on cervix. This is of no clinical significance.

uterus. If very large, they may cause pressure effects on the bladder or bowel and in pregnancy may cause obstructed labour (see Ch. 2).

Endocervical polyp

Endocervical polyps may be asymptomatic or associated with intermenstrual or postcoital bleeding. They are benign and develop from hyperplastic cervical epithelium. They are usually single, less than 1 cm and are seen as an echogenic area within the cervix (Fig. 8.19). The polyp may prolapse into the vagina. The differential diagnosis includes a pedunculated endometrial polyp or pedunculated submucosal fibroid.

Cervical carcinoma

Ultrasound imaging is not reliable for the visualisation of cervical cancer and magnetic resonance imaging is the modality of choice. Secondary effects of the tumour may be seen such as haematometra, pyometra, enlarged pelvic lymph nodes or hydronephrosis.

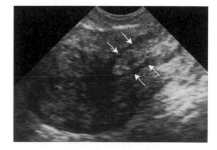

Fig. 8.19 *Endocervical polyp causing dilatation of the cervix. On speculum examination, this polyp was protruding through the external os.*

The ovaries

fertilised ovum. It normally measures 15–20 mm, is hypoechoic and has an irregular lining. Slight bleeding into the cyst frequently occurs, resulting in internal echoes or a homogenous appearance (Fig. 9.4). During the menstrual cycle the corpus luteum is rarely more than 30 mm but if conception occurs it may be much larger and rupture.

Fig. 9.4 *Typical corpus luteum measuring 15 mm, hypoechoic with very fine internal echoes.*

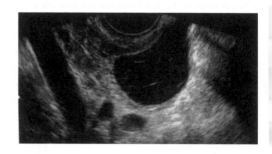

Normal ovarian appearance

During the reproductive years, follicles are normally present in the ovaries, making ultrasonic detection easy. Before the menarche and after the menopause, the ovaries are small with no visible follicles and so identification is difficult. The ovaries are oval in shape and are composed of a central medullary area with a surrounding cortical area where the follicles are generally found.

It is best to try to identify the ovaries using your transabdominal probe first. This should be done to exclude any significant enlargement. If there is a large ovarian cyst this will be seen abdominally but may be missed transvaginally as previously stated. You may not see the ovaries transabdominally and a transvaginal scan is usually necessary and better to visualise the ovaries. The technique required to locate the ovaries has already been discussed in Chapter 7. The points to recall are:

1. The ovaries are normally located medial to the internal iliac vessels but may lie anywhere in the pelvis (Fig. 9.5).

2. Measure each ovary in three dimensions, describe the appearance and record any abnormal location. The average ovarian size is $3 \times 2 \times 2$ cm.

3. You can differentiate bowel from ovary by observing peristalsis.

4. You can differentiate follicles from vessels by rotating the transducer or using colour flow.

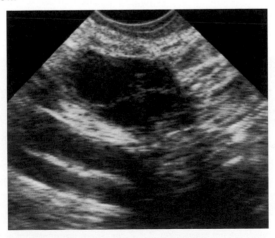

Fig. 9.5 *Right normal ovary measuring $3 \times 2.2 \times 2$ cm lying medial to the internal iliac vessels.*

Functional cysts

If a follicle fails to rupture, a *follicular cyst* may result. These are thin walled and unilocular, usually up to 4 cm in diameter. They are asymptomatic and most will be seen to regress if you repeat the scan in 6–8 weeks. Multiple follicular cysts are seen in hyperstimulated ovaries during fertility treatment.

During the menstrual cycle the corpus luteum is rarely more than 30 mm and regresses at the end of the cycle and during menstruation. If conception occurs it may be much larger. *Corpus luteal cysts* are more commonly seen in early pregnancy and may reach up to 8 cm in diameter (Fig. 2.22). They are stimulated by human chorionic gonadotrophin which has a similar action to luteinising hormone. It reaches a peak 70 days after conception and so luteal cysts regress after this time. A vascular network surrounds the cyst and occasionally haemorrhage into the cyst will occur; this may appear as debris (Fig. 9.6). Increasing tension within the cyst will cause pain and sometimes rupture with significant intraperitoneal haemorrhage.

Most functional cysts can be managed expectantly. Cyst aspiration can be undertaken in some circumstances but the risk of recurrence is high. It is important that your description is clear, stating that the cyst is unilocular with no solid components, no nodules on the wall and no internal blood flow. Always consider the differential diagnosis. In the non-pregnant patient a repeat scan in 3 months is appropriate and most cysts will have regressed. A normal CA-125 blood level will give added assurance. If you detect a functional cyst in early pregnancy, a repeat scan at 14 weeks is appropriate because many will have regressed by this time.

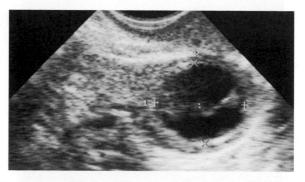

Fig. 9.6 *Corpus luteum measuring 2 × 2 cm. There were internal echoes in keeping with bleeding into the cyst. The patient was asymptomatic.*

Polycystic ovaries

Polycystic ovaries (PCO) are seen ultrasonically in about 20% of women of reproductive age. This finding alone does not mean that the woman has the polycystic ovarian syndrome (PCOS). This has been associated with hirsutism, obesity, oligomenorrhoea and infertility. In this condition, many of the ovarian follicles fail to mature and ovulate and become atrophic. This results in enlarged spherical ovaries, with echogenic stroma comparable to myometrium and numerous small cysts arranged peripherally and throughout the stroma (Fig. 9.7). The condition has been previously overdiagnosed and agreed criteria have recently been established (Rotterdam Consensus Group 2003; see Box 9.1).

1. Identify each ovary in turn using transvaginal ultrasound, as described in Chapter 7.

2. Measure in centimetres the length, width and anteroposterior (AP) diameter and take prints of images. Calculate the volume using the formula, volume (cm^3) = length × width × AP diameter × 0.53.

3. Count the number of follicles in the longitudinal and anteroposterior planes and report if 12 and more or less than 12.

4. State if there are multiple peripheral cysts.

Box 9.1 Polycystic ovarian syndrome

Two or more of the following criteria must be met:

- Oligomenorrhoea or anovulation
- Clinical and/or biochemical signs of hyperandrogenism
- PCO morphology (volume more than 10 ml; 12 or more follicles in longitudinal and anteroposterior diameter; multiple peripheral 2–9 mm cysts)

From Rotterdam Consensus Group 2003 Human Reproduction 2004; 19(1):41–47

Case Scenario (Fig. 9.7 A,B)

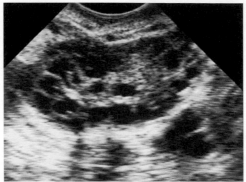

(A) Longitudinal section of right ovary.

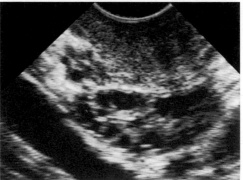

(B) Transverse section of right ovary.

The patient was a 25-year-old nulliparous woman who suffered from oligomenorrhoea. A transvaginal ultrasound of each ovary revealed more than 12 small 2–4 mm cysts scattered throughout an echogenic stroma and arranged peripherally. The illustrated right ovary measured $3.8 \times 2.7 \times 2.2$ cm, giving a volume measurement of 12 cm³ or 12 ml. This is in keeping with PCO morphology. Having also the clinical symptom of oligomenorrhoea, there are two criteria met to allow the diagnosis of the polycystic ovarian syndrome.

Abnormal ovarian appearance – benign or malignant?

Ovarian cysts present clinically in different ways (Box 9.2).

Box 9.2 Clinical presentation of ovarian cyst

Asymptomatic pelvic or abdominal mass
Pain due to:
— torsion
— rupture
— haemorrhage
— infection

It is often difficult to know whether abnormal ovarian appearances are in keeping with benign or malignant change. Germ cell tumours are more common in childhood and adolescence, functional cysts in the reproductive years and malignant tumours in perimenopausal and postmenopausal women. An abnormality will be seen with ultrasound but the exact diagnosis cannot be made until there is histological confirmation. There are certain characteristics which will raise your index of suspicion.

Malignant ovarian cysts tend be multilocular, have solid areas within the cyst and have thicker walls with nodular projections (Fig. 9.8). If there is ascites the likelihood of malignancy is high. There is no correlation between the size of an ovarian cyst and malignancy. The risk of malignancy index is based on CA-125 level, menopausal status and ultrasound findings. CA-125 is raised in 80% of ovarian cancers but can be raised with benign cysts and endometriosis. The findings considered abnormal are multilocularity, solid areas, bilateral lesions, ascites and intra-abdominal metastasis. No routine place for Doppler has been found because increased blood flow may occur in both benign and malignant cysts. Cyst aspiration is not recommended in postmenopausal women.

1. Measure the ovary in three dimensions if possible. If the cyst is very large you will have detected it on transabdominal imaging.

2. Measure the thickness of the wall of the cyst. More than 3 mm is more suggestive of malignancy.

3. Check the lining of the cyst to see if it is nodular with papillary projections.

4. Look at the septa dividing the locules. Numerous thick, irregular septa are more suggestive of malignancy.

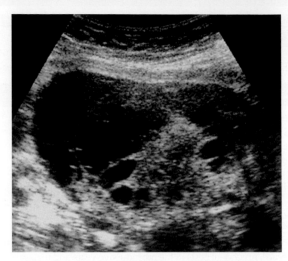

Fig. 9.8 *An 8.3 × 8.1 × 9.1 cm multilocular ovarian cyst with solid areas, some thick septa and small nodular projections. The findings were suspicious of malignancy and subsequent histology confirmed a cystadenocarcinoma of ovary.*

5. Look for solid components within the locules.

6. Check for ascites.

7. Check the other ovary. You may require to perform a transvaginal scan to do this.

8. If you suspect malignancy the patient will require further investigation and, in particular, an abdominal scan to check the liver for metastases.

Tumours of the ovary may be primary, arising from the ovary itself, or secondary, having metastasised from another site such as lung, breast, bowel or contralateral ovary. Most primary tumours are mainly cystic whereas most secondary tumours are mainly solid.

Certain characteristic appearances are specific to particular benign cysts and your understanding and knowledge of these is important.

Serous cystadenoma

This accounts for 30% of benign ovarian cysts and is the most common. Around 20% are bilateral. The average size is 10 cm but can be very large. It can be unilocular or multilocular. It contains serous fluid and so is ultrasonically anechoic. It is thin walled and has thin septations. If unilocular it has similar appearances to a follicular cyst. There should be no mural nodules (Fig. 9.9). Numerous papillary projections and thicker septations suggest malignancy. Serous cystadenocarcinoma accounts for around 40% of ovarian malignancies.

Mucinous cystadenoma

This accounts for 20% of benign ovarian cysts. It tends to be unilateral. The average size is 20 cm and may fill the pelvis. It is usually multilocular with thin septations and no solid components. It contains mucin which is gelatinous and so ultrasonically has low echogenicity (Fig. 9.10).

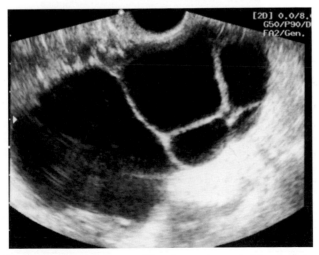

Fig. 9.9 *A 9.4 × 5.1 × 6.2 cm multilocular ovarian cyst. It is anechoic with no solid areas. The capsule appears thin, as do the septa, and there are no mural projections. The findings are suggestive of a benign cyst and subsequent histology revealed a benign cystadenoma.*

Case Scenario (Fig. 9.10)

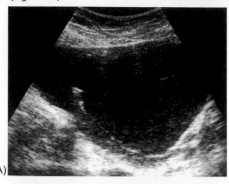

(A)

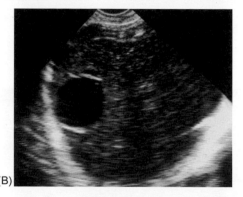

(B)

The patient was a 39-year-old nulliparous patient with a history of involuntary infertility. She was referred to the gynaecology outpatient department with a history of urinary frequency and occasional incontinence. A mass was felt arising out of the pelvis. On transabdominal scan **(A)** a 13 × 9.4 × 8 cm bilocular mass was seen. On transvaginal scan **(B)** the cyst appeared hypoechoic and there was a separate locule within the larger locule. The septa were thin and there were no solid components. The appearances were in keeping with a benign mucinous cystadenoma which was later confirmed histologically.

Dermoid (benign teratoma)

This is the most common benign ovarian cyst in younger women. It accounts for 25% of benign cysts and 20% are bilateral. The average size is around 10 cm but may be as small as 0.5 cm. It is usually unilocular and is filled with fatty sebum. Being a germ cell tumour, it may contain fat, hair, teeth or bone and these are usually contained in a solid mass of tissue projecting into the cavity of the cyst. The ultrasonic appearances vary from a diffuse echogenic mass to a cystic lesion with solid areas projecting into the lumen (Figs 9.11, 9.12). Due to the high fat content, distal acoustic shadowing will be seen. Magnetic resonance imaging can conclusively diagnose a dermoid.

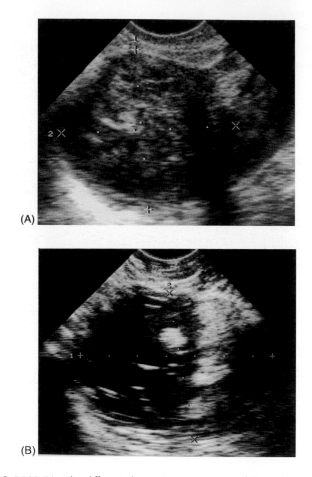

(A)

(B)

Fig. 9.11(A,B) *The different ultrasonic appearances of dermoid cysts. In **(A)** there is a diffuse echogenic mass measuring 6 × 4 × 4 cm. Histology revealed a cavity filled with yellow sebaceous material admixed with hair. In **(B)** the 7 × 7 × 8 cm mass is cystic with solid areas and looks suspicious. However, the lesion was benign and on section contained yellow sebaceous material and on one part of the wall there was a bony mass incorporating teeth.*

Case Scenario (Fig. 9.12)

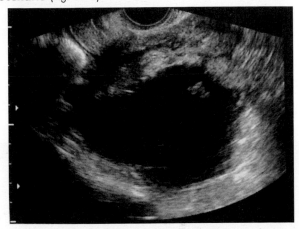

This 41-year-old woman presented with a history of menorrhagia and on vaginal examination a right adnexal mass was felt. On transvaginal scanning the uterus and left ovary appeared normal but there was a 7 × 8 × 6 cm right unilocular ovarian cyst which contained solid areas projecting into the cavity. The patient had a laparotomy and frozen section was undertaken in theatre which revealed a benign lesion, with features in keeping with a dermoid. The patient had been previously counselled and in view of her age and symptoms a total abdominal hysterectomy and bilateral salpingo-oophorectomy were undertaken.

Endometrioma

This may be an isolated finding or associated with extensive pelvic endometriosis which will not be detected ultrasonically. The average size of an endometrioma is 5 cm and it contains altered brown blood, giving rise to the term 'chocolate cyst'. It may be bilateral. Ultrasonically it is identifiable as a thick-walled, unilocular cyst containing uniform low level echoes (Fig. 9.13). If there is extensive endometriosis obliterating the pouch of Douglas, the uterus may be retroverted due to adhesions.

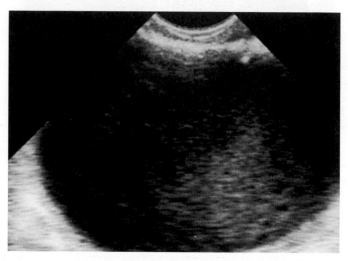

Fig. 9.13 *An 8 × 5.5 × 6 cm left-sided unilocular ovarian cyst containing uniform low level echoes in keeping with an endometrioma. Subsequent histology confirmed this.*

Fibroma

This may occur occur at any age. Although a rarer benign tumour, it can easily be confused with a fibroid, being solid and visualised as a homogeneous, hypoechoic adnexal mass (Fig. 9.14). Cystic degeneration can occur. Although benign, it can be associated with weight loss, ascites and pleural effusions (Meig's syndrome).

Case Scenario (Fig. 9.14)

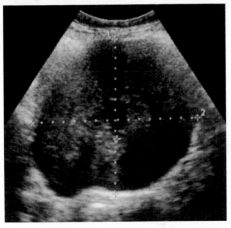

A 9.5 × 9.6 × 10 cm solid ovarian cyst with a central echo-free area in keeping with degenerative change. Histology revealed a benign fibroma with central haemorrhagic degeneration.

Peritoneal inclusion cysts

These occur after pelvic inflammatory disease or after surgery, either gynaecological or bowel. They are caused by pelvic adhesions causing fluid entrapment and may involve the ovary (Fig. 9.15). The patient may be asymptomatic or have pain. Ultrasonically they are seen as complex, irregular-shaped, multicystic masses of varying sizes.

Try to make gynaecological ultrasound a little easier for yourself by thinking of the differential diagnosis of a cystic lesion (Box 9.3) or a solid lesion (Box 9.4).

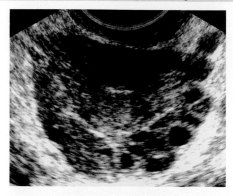

Fig. 9.15 *This transvaginal scan was taken from a 25-year-old nulliparous patient who had had a panproctocolectomy for Crohn's disease. It shows both ovaries embedded in the pouch of Douglas. One of the ovaries shows multiple small cysts and it is likely that pelvic adhesions are preventing follicular rupture.*

Box 9.3 Differential diagnosis of an adnexal cystic lesion

Functional cyst
— follicular
— corpus luteal
Hyperstimulated ovary
Cystadenoma
Distended fallopian tube
— hydrosalpinx
— pyosalpinx
Ectopic pregnancy
Endometrioma

Embryological cyst
— fimbrial
— para-ovarian
— peritoneal
— broad ligament
Peritoneal inclusion cysts (previous surgery)
Bowel
— dilated loop
— inflammatory bowel disease

Certain pathologies have very similar appearances. Make gynaecological ultrasound easy by describing your findings rather than trying to make an

Box 9.4 Differential diagnosis of a solid pelvic mass

Fibroid
Ovarian tumour
— fibroma
— secondary

Abscess
Pelvic kidney
Retroperitoneal tumour

absolute diagnosis. You can describe your findings *as suspicious of* or *in keeping with* a specific diagnosis.

Checklist for an ovarian cyst

Measure in three dimensions
Unilocular or multilocular
Solid components
Cyst wall thickness
Nodules or projections of lining
Septal thickness and regularity
Contralateral ovary
Ascites

Points to remember

1. Malignant cysts tend to be multilocular, and have solid areas and thicker walls with nodular projections.
2. The exact diagnosis of an ovarian mass will only be made after histological confirmation.
3. Think of the differential diagnosis.

The use of ultrasound for fertility problems

Investigation

When investigating a couple with fertility problems it is important to establish if the woman is ovulating, that the uterus and fallopian tubes are normal and that the woman's partner is producing normal sperm. Ultrasound, in particular transvaginal ultrasound, has proved an invaluable aid to check the female pelvic anatomy for pathology which may impair fertility. A knowledge of the previous chapters is essential because any gynaecological problem may be encountered. The following is a summary of the relevant issues.

A baseline transvaginal scan of the female pelvis should be undertaken to establish normality.

1. Identify the uterus as previously described. You should measure it to exclude hypoplasia or significant enlargement. It measures approximately 6–8 cm in length, 5 cm transversely and 4 cm anteroposteriorly. The measurements are 1–2 cm more in parous women. Scrutinise the myometrium for fibroids. Submucosal fibroids are frequently associated with fertility problems. Check the outline of the cavity to exclude any congenital abnormality, such as a bicornuate uterus (Fig. 8.14). If the scan is undertaken between days 10 and 12 of the menstrual cycle, a triple layer of endometrium should be seen measuring at least 7 mm (Fig. 8.7). It is necessary to have a minimal endometrial thickness (7 mm) to ensure successful implantation.

2. Check each adnexum in turn to identify any tubal problems. Normally the fallopian tubes cannot be visualised unless they contain fluid (hydrosalpinx) (Fig. 10.1) or pus (pyosalpinx). Both these conditions may affect a woman's fertility. Although the fallopian tubes cannot be visualised it does not mean that they are normal. Routine ultrasound will not determine if the tubes are patent. However, it is possible with ultrasound to establish tubal patency. A commercially available contrast agent comprising monosaccharide microparticles is introduced into the uterine cavity to outline the uterus and fallopian tubes. It is possible to visualise the contrast medium spilling out through the fimbrial ends thus establishing patency. Complete visualisation of the tubes is not always possible using a contrast medium and colour Doppler may be used to improve imaging. It is normally undertaken as an outpatient procedure, replacing hysterosalpingography or laparoscopy and dye as a first line of investigation.

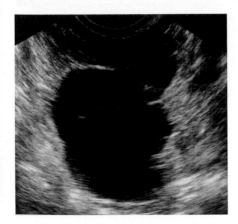

Fig. 10.1 *Characteristic appearance of a hydrosalpinx. Note the upper narrower part and the dilated fimbriated end.*

3. After establishing that there is no hydro- or pyosalpinx, the next step is to assess each ovary in turn. Move the transducer laterally to visualise the iliac vessels and the ovaries medial to them. Remember to rotate your transducer 45 degrees outwardly to bring the ovaries into view (see pp. 208–209).

In women of childbearing age the ovarian volume is 4.1–5.7 cm³. When scanning a normal ovary it is usual to see four or five follicles depending on where the woman is in her menstrual cycle (Fig. 9.5). At ovulation the dominant follicle can have a mean diameter of 21 mm (range 17–27 mm). It is therefore useful to measure the ovaries, and note the number of and measure the follicles, taking into account the phase of the menstrual cycle. If no follicles are visualised then this should be noted. After ovulation, collapse of the dominant follicle is noted and a cystic structure will be seen in the ovary. This is the corpus luteum (Fig. 9.1).

Sometimes when scanning the ovaries multiple peripheral follicles will be seen on the ovaries. The appearance may be suggestive of polycystic ovaries (Fig. 9.7). It is important to differentiate between polycystic and multifollicular ovaries. In the latter the ovary is normal in size or slightly increased and there are six or more follicles throughout ovarian stroma measuring 4–10 mm in diameter.

Checklist for ultrasound assessment for fertility

Uterus for position, size, anomalies
Endometrium (thickness, morphology)
Ovaries (assess normality and exclude polycystic ovaries)
Fallopian tubes (exclude hydrosalpinx)
Pouch of Douglas (presence of free fluid)

Assisted conception

In women with fertility problems there are a variety of treatment options depending on the underlying cause of the fertility problem.

In an assisted conception programme ultrasound is used to monitor the response of both the ovaries and the endometrium in response to hormonal treatment.

1. Ovulation monitoring may be undertaken to exclude anovulation, to time intercourse and to time intrauterine insemination.

2. During ovulation induction with clomiphene, the ovaries can be observed with ultrasound. The scan on day 8 is important to assess that there are no more than two dominant follicles. Intercourse can thus be timed. If there are more than two follicles the cycle should be cancelled.

3. During superovulation, ovarian scanning is essential to aim for no more than two follicles of 17 mm, after which luteinising hormone can be safely given.

4. During the in vitro fertilisation cycle, ultrasound is used to track follicular development. Three follicles sized 17 mm or more are induced and oocytes retrieved by needle aspiration (Fig. 10.2). Great care must be taken to distinguish a follicle from the internal iliac vessels, and colour flow Doppler is helpful in this respect.

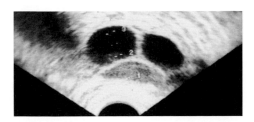

Fig. 10.2 *Follicles about to be aspirated for oocyte retrieval. Note the centimetre gauged needle biopsy track lines. It is common practice by reproductive medicine specialists to invert the image as shown. This is helpful because the needle will then appear from the inferior margin in the same direction as insertion.*

We are now at the boundary zone of *Gynaecological Ultrasound Made Easy* and should stop here!

Further reading

Bates J 1997 Practical gynaecological ultrasound. Oxford University Press, Oxford

Bianchi DW, Crombleholme TM, D'Alton ME 2000 Fetology: diagnosis and management of the fetal patient. McGraw-Hill, New York

Bisset RAL, Khan AN, Thomas NB 2002 Differential diagnosis in obstetric and gynaecologic ultrasound. Saunders, Philadelphia

Bourne T, Valentin L 2004 Ultrasound in gynaecology. In: Arulkumaran S (ed.) Clinical obstetrics and gynaecology, Vol 18, No. 1. Baillière Tindall, London

Callen PW 2000 Ultrasonography in obstetrics and gynaecology, 4th edn. Saunders, Philadelphia

Chudleigh T, Thilaganathan B 2004 Obstetric ultrasound: how, why and when, 3rd edn. Elsevier, London

Dewbury K, Meire H, Cosgrove D, Farrant P 2001 Ultrasound in obstetrics and gynaecology. Clinical ultrasound – a comprehensive text. Vol 3, 2nd edn. Churchill Livingstone, London

Doubilet PM, Benson C 2003 Atlas of ultrasound in obstetrics and gynecology: a multimedia reference. Lippincott Williams & Wilkins, Philadelphia

Fleischer AC 2004 Sonography in gynaecology and obstetrics: just the facts. McGraw-Hill, New York

Hricak H, Reinhold C, Ascher SM 2004 Pocket radiologist: gynaecology – top 100 diagnoses. Saunders, Philadelphia

Johnson PT, Kurtz AB 2001 Case review: obstetric and gynecologic ultrasound. Mosby, St Louis

Kremkau FW 2002 Diagnostic ultrasound. Principles and instruments, 6th edn. Saunders, Philadelphia

Lees C, Deane C, Albaiges G 2003 Making sense of obstetric Doppler ultrasound. Arnold, London

Nyberg DA, McGahan JP, Pretorius DH, Pilu G 2003 Diagnostic imaging of fetal abnormalities. Lippincott Williams & Wilkins, Philadelphia

Sanders RC 2002 Structural fetal abnormalities: the total picture, 2nd edn. Mosby, St Louis

Woodward PJ, Kennedy A, Sohaey R 2003 Pocket radiologist: obstetrics – top 100 diagnoses. Saunders, Philadelphia

Cochrane Reviews (search on internet for Cochrane Collaboration)

Biophysical profile for fetal assessment in high risk pregnancies
Doppler ultrasound for fetal assessment in high risk pregnancies
Instruments for chorionic villus sampling for prenatal diagnosis
Routine Doppler ultrasound in pregnancy
Routine ultrasound in late pregnancy (after 24 weeks)
Ultrasound for fetal assessment in early pregnancy

Good medical practice documents from the Royal College of Obstetricians and Gynaecologists (available from www.rcog.org.uk)

Amniocentesis
Early pregnancy loss – management
Investigation and management of endometriosis
Investigation and management of the small for gestational age fetus
Ovarian cysts in postmenopausal women
Placenta praevia – diagnosis and management
Trophoblastic disease
Tubal pregnancies

SIGN (Scottish Intercollegiate Guidelines Network) (www.sign.ac.uk)

Investigation of postmenopausal bleeding (61) September 2002

Working party reports

Down syndrome screening programme information (RCOG)
Routine ultrasound scanning before 24 weeks of pregnancy. Health Technology Assessment Advice 5 (NHS Quality Improvement Scotland)
Ultrasound screening (from www.rcog.org.uk) July 2000

Index

Note: page numbers in *italics* refer to figures and tables.